National Health Issues

Series Editor: Cara Acred

Volume 251

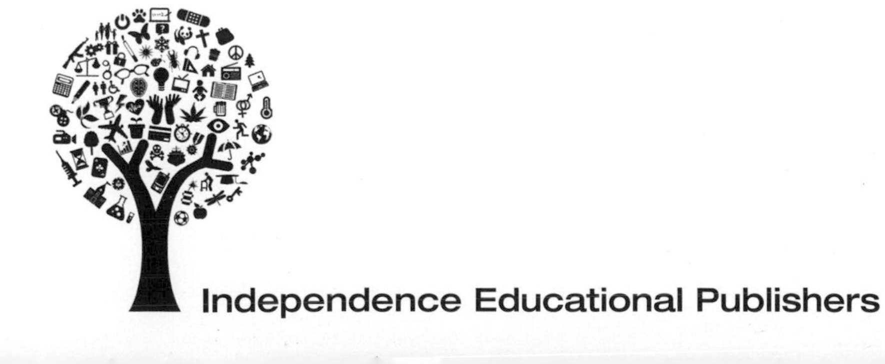
Independence Educational Publishers

First published by Independence Educational Publishers
The Studio, High Green
Great Shelford
Cambridge CB22 5EG
England

British Library Cataloguing in Publication Data

National health issues. -- (Issues ; 251)
1. Great Britain. National Health Service. 2. Medical policy--Great Britain. 3. Public health--Great Britain.
I. Series II. Acred, Cara editor of compilation.
362.1'0941-dc23

ISBN-13: 9781861686572

Printed in Great Britain

MWL Print Group Ltd

Contents

Chapter 1: What is the NHS?

Chapter 2: Healthcare problems

Chapter 3: The future of the NHS

Introduction

National Health Issues is Volume 251 in the ***ISSUES*** series. The aim of the series is to offer current, diverse information about important issues in our world, from a UK perspective.

ABOUT NATIONAL HEALTH ISSUES

The NHS is a constant victim of scrutiny; politicians, press and public regularly voice their opinions on its successes and failures, meaning that separating 'spin' from fact is often next-to impossible. As the NHS reaches 65-years-old, should we be celebrating its achievements or mourning its mistakes? What is the current state of care in our hospitals? What will our health service look like in ten years' time? National Health Issues explores all of these questions and more.

OUR SOURCES

Titles in the ***ISSUES*** series are designed to function as educational resource books, providing a balanced overview of a specific subject.

The information in our books is comprised of facts, articles and opinions from many different sources, including:

- Newspaper reports and opinion pieces
- Website factsheets
- Magazine and journal articles
- Statistics and surveys
- Government reports
- Literature from special interest groups

A NOTE ON CRITICAL EVALUATION

Because the information reprinted here is from a number of different sources, readers should bear in mind the origin of the text and whether the source is likely to have a particular bias when presenting information (or when conducting their research). It is hoped that, as you read about the many aspects of the issues explored in this book, you will critically evaluate the information presented.

It is important that you decide whether you are being presented with facts or opinions. Does the writer give a biased or unbiased report? If an opinion is being expressed, do you agree with the writer? Is there potential bias to the 'facts' or statistics behind an article?

ASSIGNMENTS

In the back of this book, you will find a selection of assignments designed to help you engage with the articles you have been reading and to explore your own opinions. Some tasks will take longer than others and there is a mixture of design, writing and research based activities that you can complete alone or in a group.

FURTHER RESEARCH

At the end of each article we have listed its source and a website that you can visit if you would like to conduct your own research. Please remember to critically evaluate any sources that you consult and consider whether the information you are viewing is accurate and unbiased.

Useful weblinks

www.bma.org.uk

www.health.org.uk

www.keepournhspublic.com

www.midstaffspublicinquiry.com

www.moneyadviceservice.org.uk

www.nhs.uk

www.nuffieldtrust.org

Chapter 1

What is the NHS?

About the National Health Service (NHS)

Since its launch in 1948, the NHS has grown to become the world's largest publicly funded health service. It is also one of the most efficient, most egalitarian and most comprehensive.

The NHS was born out of a long-held ideal that good healthcare should be available to all, regardless of wealth, a principle that remains at its core. With the exception of some charges, such as prescriptions and optical and dental services, the NHS remains free at the point of use for anyone who is resident in the UK. That is currently more than 63.2 million people. It covers everything from antenatal screening and routine treatments for long-term conditions, to transplants, emergency treatment and end-of-life care.

Responsibility for healthcare in Northern Ireland, Scotland and Wales is devolved to the Northern Ireland Assembly, the Scottish Government and the Welsh Assembly Government, respectively.

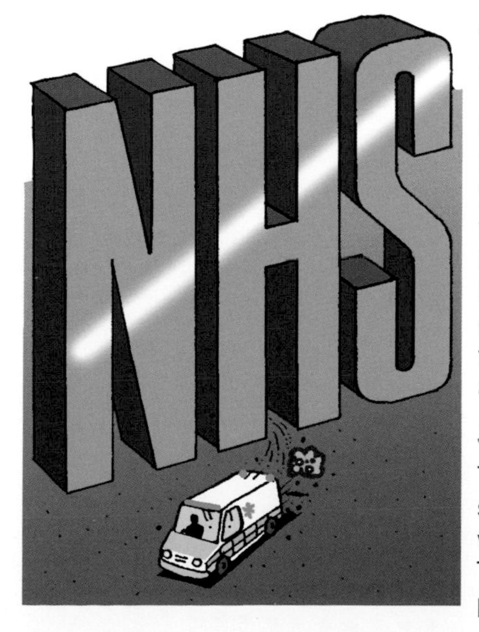

Scale

The NHS employs more than 1.7 million people. Of those, just under half are clinically qualified, including, 39,780 general practitioners (GPs), 370,327 nurses, 18,687 ambulance staff and 105,711 hospital and community health service (HCHS) medical and dental staff.

Only the Chinese People's Liberation Army, the Wal-Mart supermarket chain and the Indian Railways directly employ more people.

The NHS in England is the biggest part of the system by far, catering to a population of 53 million and employing more than 1.35 million people. The NHS in Scotland, Wales and Northern Ireland employs 153,427, 84,817 and 78,000 people, respectively.

The NHS deals with over one million patients every 36 hours.

Funding

Funding for the NHS comes directly from taxation and is granted to the Department of Health by Parliament. When the NHS was launched in 1948 it had a budget of £437 million (roughly £9 billion at today's value). For 2012/2013 it is around £108.9 billion.

Structure

The NHS in England is undergoing some big changes, most of which will take effect on 1 April 2013. This will include the abolition of primary care trusts (PCTs) and strategic health authorities (SHAs) and the introduction of clinical commissioning groups (CCGs) and Healthwatch England.

However, none of this will have an effect on how you access front-line services and your healthcare will remain free at the point of use. For detailed information about all the changes, see the section about the NHS structure.

Performance

In the UK, life expectancy has been rising and infant mortality has been falling since the NHS was established. Both figures compare favourably with other nations. Surveys also show that patients are generally satisfied with the care they receive from the NHS. Importantly, people who have had recent direct experience of the NHS tend to report being more satisfied than people who have not.

In 2010, the Commonwealth Fund declared that in comparison with the healthcare systems of six other countries (Australia, Canada, Germany, The Netherlands, New Zealand and USA) the NHS was the second most impressive overall. The NHS was rated as the best system in terms of efficiency, effective care and cost-related problems. It was also ranked second for patient equality and safety.

28 January 2013

⇨ The above information is reprinted with kind permission from NHS Choices. Please visit www.nhs.uk for further information.

The history of the NHS in England

5 July 1948 – The NHS is born

When health secretary Aneurin Bevan opens Park Hospital in Manchester, it is the climax of a hugely ambitious plan to bring good healthcare to all. For the first time, hospitals, doctors, nurses, pharmacists, opticians and dentists are brought together under one umbrella organisation to provide services that are free for all at the point of delivery.

The central principles are clear: the health service will be available to all and financed entirely from taxation, which means that people pay into it according to their means.

1952 – Charges of one shilling are introduced for prescriptions

Prescription charges of one shilling (5p) are introduced and a flat rate of £1 for ordinary dental treatment is also brought in on 1 June 1952. Prescription charges are abolished in 1965 and prescriptions remain free until June 1968, when the charges are reintroduced.

1962 – Enoch Powell's Hospital Plan

The medical profession criticises the separation of the NHS into three parts – hospitals, general practice and local health authorities – and calls for unification. The Hospital Plan approves the development of district general hospitals for population areas of about 125,000 and, in doing so, lays out a pattern for the future. The ten-year programme is new territory for the NHS and it soon becomes clear that it has underestimated the cost and time it would take to build new hospitals. However, a start is made and, with the advent of postgraduate education centres, nurses and doctors will be given a better future.

1967 – The Salmon Report

The Salmon Report is published and sets out recommendations for developing the nursing staff structure and the status of the profession in hospital management. The Cogwheel Report considers the organisation of doctors in hospitals and proposes speciality groupings. It also highlights the efforts being made to reduce the disadvantages of the three-part NHS structure – hospitals, general practice and local health authorities – acknowledging the complexity of the NHS and the importance of change to meet future needs.

1968 – Britain's first heart transplant

South Africa-born surgeon Donald Ross carries out Britain's first heart transplant at the National Heart Hospital in Marylebone, London, on 3 May 1968. Ross leads a team of 18 doctors and nurses to operate on the unnamed 45-year-old man in the seven-hour procedure. The donor was a 26-year-old labourer called Patrick Ryan. The British operation is the tenth heart transplant to be undertaken in the world. The patient dies after 46 days from an associated infection and only six transplants are carried out over the next ten years for fear of failure.

1972 – CT scans revolutionise the way doctors examine the body

Computed tomography (CT) scanners produce three-dimensional images from a large series of two-dimensional X-rays. The first one is dreamt up in England in 1967 by Godfrey Newbold Hounsfield and becomes a reality in 1972. Since that initial invention, CT scanners have developed enormously, but the principle remains the same.

1980 – Keyhole surgery

A surgeon uses a telescopic rod with fibre optic cable to remove a gallbladder. The procedure will go on to be one of the most common uses of this kind of surgery. It will also be used for hernia repairs and removal of the colon and the kidney.

1980 – Black Report

Commissioned three years earlier b David Ennals, then Secretary of State the report aims to investigate th inequality of healthcare that still exist despite the foundation of the NHS, i.e differences between the social classe in the usage of medical services, infar mortality rates and life expectancy Poor people are still more likely to di earlier than rich ones. The Whitehea Report in 1987 and the Acheso Report in 1998 reached the sam conclusions as the Black Report.

1981 – Improved health of babies

Childhood survival has bee revolutionised by vaccinatio programmes, better sanitation an improved standards of living, resultin in better health of both mother an child. Increased numbers of birth in hospital has meant that wher unexpected problems do occu medical help is on hand. Around on baby in eight requires some kind c special care following birth. 20 year ago, only 20% of babies weighing les than 1,000g (2lb 2oz) at birth survivec Now that figure is closer to 80%.

1986 – AIDS health campaign

The Government launches bigges public health campaign in history t educate people about the threat c AIDs as a result of HIV. Following number of high-profile deaths, th advertising campaign sets out t shock, with images of tombstone and icebergs, followed early in 198 by a household leaflet, 'Don't die c ignorance'.

1988 – Breast screening is introduced

To reduce breast cancer deaths i women over 50 this project is launche with breast-screening units aroun the country providing mammograms Screening, together with improve drug therapies, will help to cut breas cancer deaths by more than 20%, trend that looks set to continue.

1990 – NHS and Community Care Act

Now health authorities will manage their own budgets and buy healthcare from hospitals and other health organisations. In order to be deemed a 'provider' of such healthcare, organisations will become NHS Trusts, that is, independent organisations with their own managements.

1991 – First NHS Trusts established

57 NHS Trusts are established to make the service more responsive to the user at a local level.

1994 – NHS Organ Donor Register

The NHS Organ Donor Register is launched following a five-year campaign by John and Rosemary Cox. In 1989 their son Peter died of a brain tumour. He had asked for his organs to be used to help others. The Coxes said that there should be a register for people who wish to donate their organs.

1998 NHS Direct launches

A nurse-led advice service provides people with 24-hour health advice over the phone. This service will go on to become one of the largest single e-health services in the world, handling more than half a million calls each month.

2000 – NHS walk-in centres

New health facilities open offering convenient access, round-the-clock, 365 days a year. NHS walk-in centres are managed by Primary Care Trusts. There are around 90 centres dealing with minor illnesses and injuries.

2002 – Primary Care Trusts launched

Primary Care Trusts oversee 29,000 GPs and 21,000 NHS dentists. They are in charge of vaccination administration and control of epidemics, they also control 80 per cent of the total NHS budget. As local organisations, they are best positioned to understand the needs of their community, so they can make sure that the organisations providing health and social care services are working effectively.

2004 – Patient Choice Pilots

All patients waiting longer than six months for an operation are given a choice of an alternative place of treatment. Everyone who is referred by their doctor for hospital treatment is given a choice of at least four hospitals.

2008 – Free choice is introduced

Free choice is introduced on 1 April 2008. Patients can choose from any hospital or clinic that meets NHS standards. Patients who are referred by their GP for their first consultant-led outpatient appointment can choose from any hospital or clinic that meets NHS standards.

2008 – The NHS at 60

On 5 July 2008, the NHS celebrates its 60th birthday with events across the country.

2008 – HPV vaccination programme

In September 2008, a national programme to vaccinate girls aged 12 and 13 against the human papilloma virus (HPV) is launched to help prevent cervical cancer. A three-year catch-up campaign is also introduced, which will offer the HPV vaccine, also known as the cervical cancer jab, to girls who are 13- to 18-years-old.

2009 – New NHS Constitution

The NHS Constitution is published on 21 January 2009. For the first time in the history of the NHS, the Constitution brings together details of what staff, patients and the public can expect from the NHS. It aims to ensure the NHS will always do what it was set up to do in 1948: provide high-quality healthcare that's free and for everyone.

2009 – New Horizons programme launched

New Horizons brings together local and national organisations and individuals to work towards a society that values mental well-being as much as physical health.

2009 – NHS Health Checks

Primary Care Trusts begin implementing the NHS Health Check programme in April 2009. It has the potential to prevent an average of 1,600 heart attacks and strokes and save up to 650 lives each year. It could prevent over 4,000 people a year from developing diabetes and detect at least 20,000 cases of diabetes or kidney disease earlier, allowing people to manage their condition better and improving their quality of life.

2010 – The Mid Staffordshire NHS Foundation Trust public inquiry

The Mid Staffordshire inquiry is based on a previous report carried out by the Healthcare Commission (now the Care Quality Commission) in March 2009. The investigation was into the apparently high mortality rates of patients admitted as emergencies to Mid Staffordshire NHS Foundation Trust since April 2005, and the care provided to these patients.

On 9 June 2010 the then Secretary of State for Health, Andrew Lansley MP, announced a full public inquiry into the role of the commissioning, supervisory and regulatory bodies in the monitoring of Mid Staffordshire Foundation NHS Trust.

2011 – The Health and Social Care Bill

The Health and Social Care Bill was published in draft form on 19 January 2011. The Bill takes forward the *Equity and Excellence: Liberating the NHS white paper* (July 2010) and is a crucial part of the Government's vision to modernise the NHS so that it is built around patients, led by health professionals and focused on delivering world-class healthcare outcomes.

2012 – The Health and Social Care Act

The Health and Social Care Act 2012 was first published on 15 June 2012 and took effect on 1 April 2013. The Act brought in the most wide-ranging reforms of the NHS since it was founded in 1948.

It puts clinicians at the centre of commissioning, frees up providers to innovate, empowers patients and gives a new focus to public health. The Act covers the following five themes:

- ⇨ strengthening the commissioning of NHS services
- ⇨ increasing democratic accountability and public voice
- ⇨ liberating provision of NHS services
- ⇨ strengthening public health services
- ⇨ reforming health and care arm's-length bodies.

2012 – Innovation in primary care

In partnership with NHS London, the Design Council has supported London's GPs to generate and implement new ideas for improving the services they offer patients. Speakers from general practice, NHS commissioning, research, academic institutions, industry and design discussed the ever-changing primary care landscape and specific GP-centric challenges both practices and patients now face. Prevalent topics included access to GP services (use of technology and infrastructure), empowerment of patients, empowerment of GPs (networks, capitation, diffusion of innovation) and GPs' role in wider public health initiatives.

2013 – Final report into the Mid Staffordshire NHS Foundation Trust public inquiry published

Following an extensive inquiry into failings at Mid Staffordshire NHS Foundation Trust, Robert Francis QC published his final report on 6 February 2013. It highlights a whole system failure, and not just one NHS Trust. A system which should have had checks and balances in place, and have been working to ensure patients were treated with dignity and suffered no harm. The 1,782-page report has 290 recommendations which have major implications for all levels of the health service across England. This includes a more patient-centred approach, better medical training and nursing, as well as better complaints handling and service governance and regulation.

2013 – The Keogh Mortality Review

On 6 February 2013, the Prime Minister announced that he had asked Professor Sir Bruce Keogh, NHS Medical Director for England, to review the quality of care and treatment provided by those NHS Trusts and NHS Foundation Trusts that are persistent outliers on mortality indicators. A total of 14 hospital trusts are being investigated as part of this review.

2013 – The new NHS

The NHS is undergoing major changes in its core structure. The new health and care system became fully operational on 1 April 2013. It delivers the ambitions set out in the Health and Social Care Act. Public Health England, the NHS Trust Development Authority and Health Education England took on their full range of responsibilities at the same time.

NHS England is an independent body, separated from the Government. Its main aim is to improve health outcomes for people in England. It will do this by creating the culture and conditions for health and care services and staff to deliver the highest standard of care and ensure valuable public resources are used effectively to get the best outcomes for individuals, communities and society now and for future generations.

Locally, clinical commissioning groups, made up of doctors, nurses and other health professionals, buy services for patients, while local councils formally took on their new roles in promoting public health. Health and well-being boards bring together local organisations to work in partnership and Healthwatch England provides a powerful voice for patients and local communities.

2013 – Putting Patients First: The NHS England Business Plan for 2013/2014–2015/2016

Putting Patients First explains how NHS England's commitment to transparency and increasing patients' voices are fundamental to improving patient care. The plan, published in April 2013, describes an 11-point scorecard which NHS England will introduce for measuring performance of key priorities, focused on receiving direct feedback from patients, their families and NHS staff.

This supports the cultural change needed to put people at the centre of the NHS, a key theme in the report by Robert Francis QC, by making sure patients' voices are heard and used to deliver better services.

2013 – Updated version of the NHS Constitution published

An updated NHS Constitution was published on 1 April 2013, following a consultation that sought views on a number of proposed changes. Important areas that were improved include:

- ⇨ patient involvement
- ⇨ feedback
- ⇨ duty of candour
- ⇨ end of life care
- ⇨ integrated care
- ⇨ complaints
- ⇨ patient information
- ⇨ staff rights, responsibilities and commitments
- ⇨ dignity, respect and compassion.

There were also some technical amendments to ensure that the NHS Constitution is in line with the new health and care system introduced in April 2013.

2013 – The National Health Service 65th anniversary

The NHS turns 65 on 5 July 2013. We are looking back at the achievements since its launch in 1948 to highlight champions and heroes who make the health service what it is today.

⇨ The above information is reprinted with kind permission from NHS Choices. Please visit www.nhs.uk for further information.

Do you need private medical insurance?

Private medical insurance (also known as health insurance) can supplement what's available on the NHS. If you don't already have it as part of your employee benefits package and you can afford to pay the premiums, you might decide it's worth paying extra to have more choice over your care.

What is private medical insurance?

Most UK residents are entitled to free healthcare from the NHS.

Health insurance pays all – or some – of your medical bills if you are treated privately. It gives you a choice in the level of care you get and how and when it is provided.

You don't have to take out private medical insurance – but if you don't want to use the NHS, you might find it hard to pay for private treatment without insurance, especially for serious conditions.

What does private medical insurance cover?

Like all insurance, the cover you get from private medical insurance depends on the policy you buy.

Basic private medical insurance usually picks up the costs of most in-patient treatments (tests and surgery) and day-care surgery.

Some policies extend to out-patient treatments (such as specialists and consultants) and may pay you a small fixed amount for each night you spend in an NHS hospital.

What private medical insurance doesn't cover

Your insurance usually won't cover private treatment for:

- pre-existing medical conditions
- chronic illnesses such as HIV/AIDs-related illnesses, diabetes, epilepsy, hypertension and related illnesses
- normal pregnancy and childbirth costs
- organ transplants
- injuries relating to dangerous sports or arising from war or war-like hostilities
- cosmetic surgery to improve your appearance.

You may be able to choose a policy which covers mental health, depression and sports injuries but these aren't always covered.

Do you need private medical insurance?

It's very much a personal choice. You get free treatment on the NHS, so you only really need private medical insurance if:

- you want to be covered for drugs and treatment you can't get on the NHS, like specialist surgery for sports-related injuries (check that the treatment is included in your policy before you buy)
- you just don't want to use the NHS and would prefer to stick to private hospitals where possible
- you would prefer not to wait for NHS treatment.

Who doesn't need private medical insurance cover?

You don't need private medical insurance if:

- you're happy to rely on the NHS for your care
- you already have medical insurance through your employee benefits package
- you only have spare cash for basic insurance, like car and home insurance (and life insurance if you have dependants)
- you have debts to repay and no savings – you should put your money towards those, rather than private medical insurance
- you can pay for individual treatments – if you have sufficient savings it might be more cost effective to pay for any treatment you may need privately than to pay regular insurance premiums

Key facts

- **In January 2011, 11.1% of the UK population had private medical insurance.**
- **The average annual premium for private medical insurance is £1,092.**
- **Private hospitals generated revenues of around £3.8 billion in 2010.**
- **Around 2% of private hospital revenue was generated from overseas patients.**
- **There are 73 private patient units (PPUs) within NHS hospitals.**
- **NHS income from treating private patients in 2011 was £445 million.**

Source: Private Healthcare: Key Facts (February 2012), *Private Healthcare UK, 2012*

- you're worried about your child becoming sick – children get immediate priority treatment on the NHS.

Pros and cons of private medical insurance

Note: all of this depends on the type of policy you buy.

Pros

- Specialist referrals. You can ask your GP to refer you to an expert or specialist working privately to get a second opinion or specialist treatment.
- Get the scans you want. If the NHS delays a scan, or won't let you have one, you can use your cover to pay for it.
- Reduce the waiting time. You can use your insurance to reduce the time you spend waiting for NHS treatment if your wait time is more than six weeks.
- Choose your surgeon and hospital. You can (in theory) choose a surgeon and hospital to suit your time and place – which isn't possible on the NHS.
- Get a private room. You can use it to get a private room, rather than staying in an open ward which might be mixed-sex.
- Specialist drugs and treatments may be available. Some specialist drugs and treatments aren't available on the NHS because they're too expensive or not approved by the National Institute for Health and Clinical Excellence in England and Wales (NICE) or the Scottish Medicines Consortium (SMC).
- Physiotherapy. You get quicker access to physiotherapy sessions if you have insurance than you would through NHS treatment.

Cons

- You might get better care on the NHS. If you have a serious illness such as cancer, heart disease or a stroke, you'll get priority NHS treatment. NHS hospitals can be as good as, or better, than private hospitals.
- It's expensive – and the price will go up. A typical family premium (two adults in their 40s and two children under ten) can vary from £700 to £1,650 per year. Premiums will rise every year, and with age – so by the time you're older, and more likely to need hospital treatment, you may not be able to afford it.
- Chronic illnesses aren't usually covered. Most policies don't cover chronic illnesses which are incurable, such as diabetes and some cancers.
- There may not be any local treatment options. If you choose a policy with an approved list of consultants and hospitals this may not include the expert consultant you want to see or a convenient location for treatment.

Is private medical insurance good value for money?

Waiting times in the NHS are currently pretty good and fairly stable, so there's less need to pay privately in order to reduce the time it takes you to get back to work or to good health.

It can be good value if you might need specialist, expensive treatment. If you're a sporting enthusiast, for example, you might want access to specialist private treatment that isn't available in the NHS – like surgeons and experts who only do private work. You'd need to have a policy that covers the type of treatment you might need.

If you needed to make more than one claim, it's quite likely that private medical insurance would save you money.

Even if you get private medical insurance, you will keep your right to use the NHS. It remains a safety net that will pick up the tab for anything that isn't covered by your insurance policy.

Alternative options if you want to go private

- Use savings for all or part of your medical costs – around one in five private patients do this. Hip and knee replacements cost an average of £10,000 each, while MRI scans cost from £600. You can shop around for scan prices – your GP can help you do this.
- Just pay for a private consultation if you want an expert or second opinion. Then, if necessary, your consultant will refer you back into the NHS for treatment.

Other types of insurance to consider

If you fall ill or have an accident and can't work, you might find it hard to keep up mortgage payments or handle the bills – especially if you don't have enough savings or sick pay from your employer. Your priority should be insurance that keeps you out of financial difficulty such as income protection.

- The above information is reprinted with kind permission from The Money Advice Service. Please visit www.moneyadviceservice.co.uk for further information.

the Money Advice Service

Patients with private medical insurance cost the NHS millions

Patients with private medical insurance have the comfort of knowing that if they fall ill they can receive the best treatment in the best surroundings. So why do a significant proportion of privately insured patients decide to seek treatment from the NHS instead?

A report by private health analysts Laing and Buisson estimates that almost one in three patients receiving care in an NHS hospital is privately insured. While these patients could opt to have their insurance companies pay for the treatment they need, it seems that many are worried about the repercussions of doing so. Many private health policies enforce a significant excess charge when a claim is submitted and patients are also concerned that their premium will be negatively affected. Some insurers even offer patients cash payments if they choose NHS treatment.

It is estimated that the NHS performs 250,000 operations each year on patients with private medical insurance, costing a total of £359 million. In addition to which, £609 million is spent on emergency medical treatment. Private medical insurance does not cover emergency care but can be used to pay for after-care such as physiotherapy.

The report from Laing and Buisson was commissioned by HCA International, which owns six private hospitals in London. Their Commercial Director, Keith Biddlestone, said: 'Private healthcare is about choice and many patients choose to move between private and NHS care – but these figures show just how hard private medical insurers rely on the NHS to maintain profitability.'

With the NHS spending a total of £968 million each year treating patients who have private medical insurance, what would happen if all of these patients decided to 'go-private' instead? Would the private medical industry cope or crumble?

1 August 2012

⇨ The above information is reprinted with kind permission from Independence Educational Publishers.

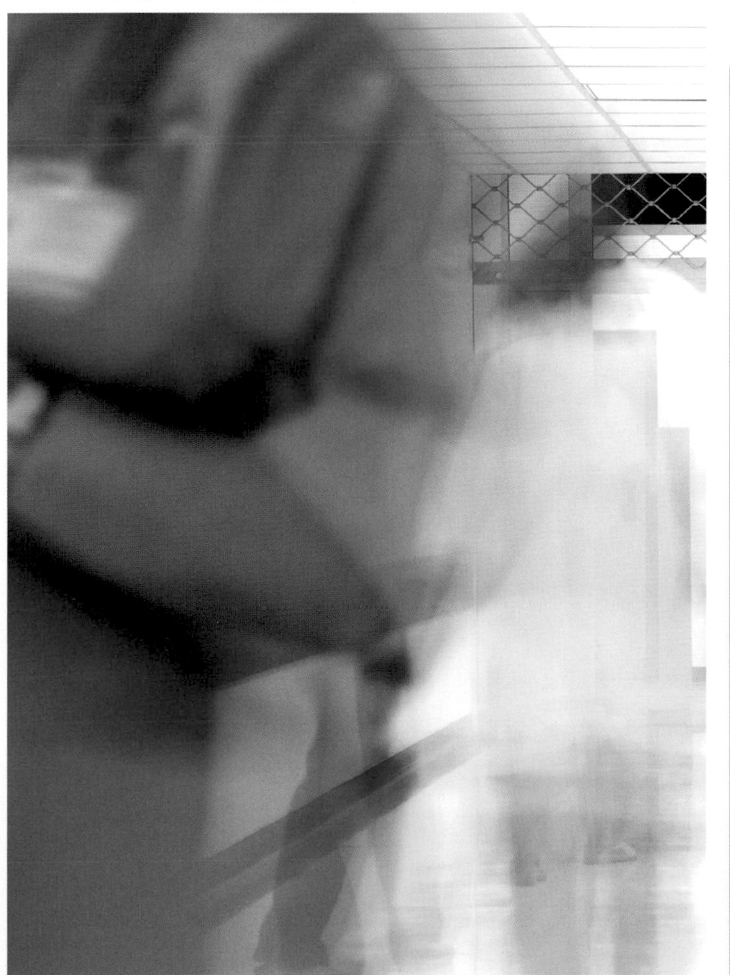

NHS versus private

- **73% consider the NHS to be one of the UK's greatest achievements.**
- **41% of people in the UK think that the health service as it exists today is unlikely to last until 2020.**
- **22% think is will survive in its current form.**
- **61% think that patients should be able to get treated at private hospitals for NHS prices where capacity permits.**
- **35% believe that opening the NHS to competition from the private sector will increase levels of care.**
- **53% of people would pay for private healthcare if they could afford it.**

Source: Healthcare: NHS versus private, *YouGov plc., 2013*

How does the NHS compare?

By Rita O'Brien

Much of the current public discussion about the NHS, particularly during the passage of the Health & Social Care Act, is ill-informed, and often merely repeats government propaganda. This aims to convince people that the NHS is failing, in order to justify their destructive changes. The real story about the NHS is very different. The information below is taken from independent, international studies, which looked at the delivery of healthcare in the major western countries, and the NHS comes out looking very good!

How effective is the NHS?

The NHS was ranked first in terms of access to healthcare, with ability to pay not being an issue. This is often ignored, because we are now so used to being able to go to our doctor. But for many countries, this is a problem – the most extreme being the USA, where over 40 million people have no access to regular healthcare because they cannot afford health insurance.

There are problems in the NHS – need for improvements in waiting lists and care for the elderly. But even when these issues are included, research rates the NHS as second only to The Netherlands in effectiveness of care delivery.

How good is NHS care?

A major part of the anti-NHS propaganda has been that it delivers worse treatment than our European neighbours (particularly France), with poorer outcomes. This is contradicted by research. Heart Disease Between 1980 and 2006, the UK had the largest fall in death rates in Europe, and by this year, would have a lower death rate than France.

Breast Cancer Death rates in the UK have fallen by 40% over the past 30 years, closing the gap with France.

Lung Cancer Death rates amongst men have fallen since 1979, and are now lower than those in France. This may of course be more linked to men smoking less!

Much of the debate about treatment in the NHS has been fuelled by those hostile to it, cherry-picking statistics rather than celebrating its achievements!

Also data across countries are not uniform. For example, French data covers only 15% of cancer patients, whereas UK covers 100%.

How much does the NHS cost?

Much of the justification for the changes to the NHS has been that it is too expensive – trying to persuade people that 'we cannot afford it'. The opposite is the case.

We spend less of our total GDP on health (8%) than comparable western countries: Germany (10.5%), France (11.2%) and the USA (16%).

Our management costs are lower than most; in 2009 we used 1.5% of our total health budget, compared with France (6.8%) and the USA (7%).

This means we made all those improvements in health outcomes, even though we spent far less on healthcare than most other countries. A study of cancer mortality rates in 2011 found that the NHS achieved major reductions in deaths on proportionately less money than the nine largest EU countries and the USA. The NHS gets more healthcare from every £ we spend!

The move to a market-based, privately-provided, system would send us in the opposite direction, towards the USA. This would make healthcare more expensive and would make it less affordable! All these changes are ideologically driven and have nothing to do with how effective and cost efficient the NHS is.

November 2012

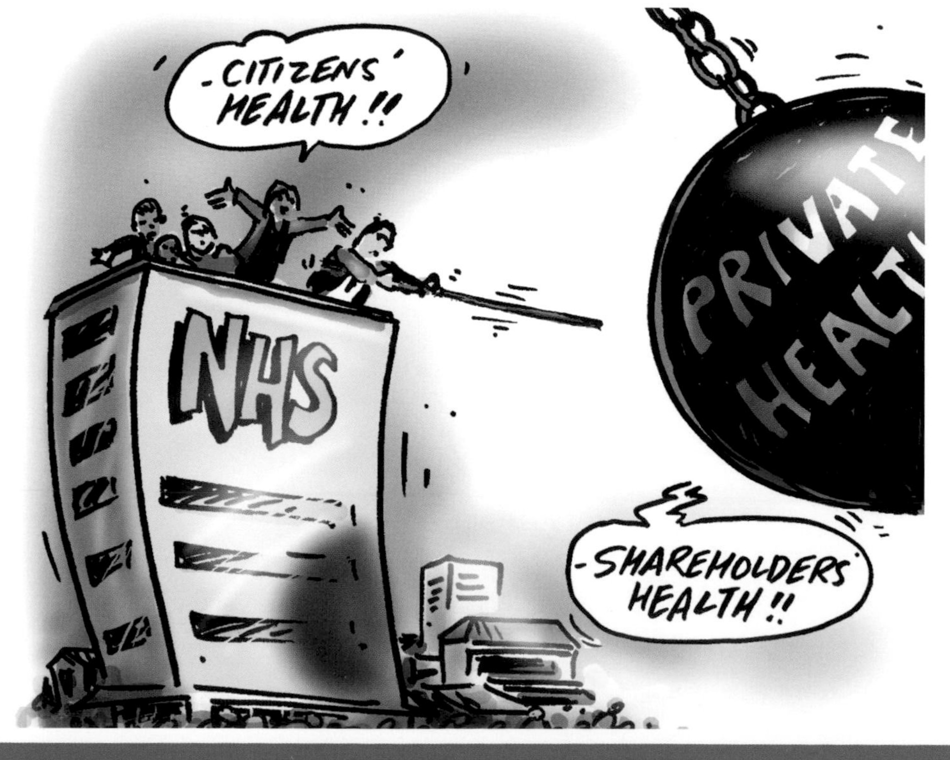

References

The Commonwealth Fund 2010 International Health Policy Survey

John Appleby, *Does Poor Health Justify NHS Reform?*, British Medical Journal, January 21, 2011

⇨ The above information is reprinted with kind permission from East Kent Keep Our NHS Public. Please visit www.keepournhspublic.com for further information.

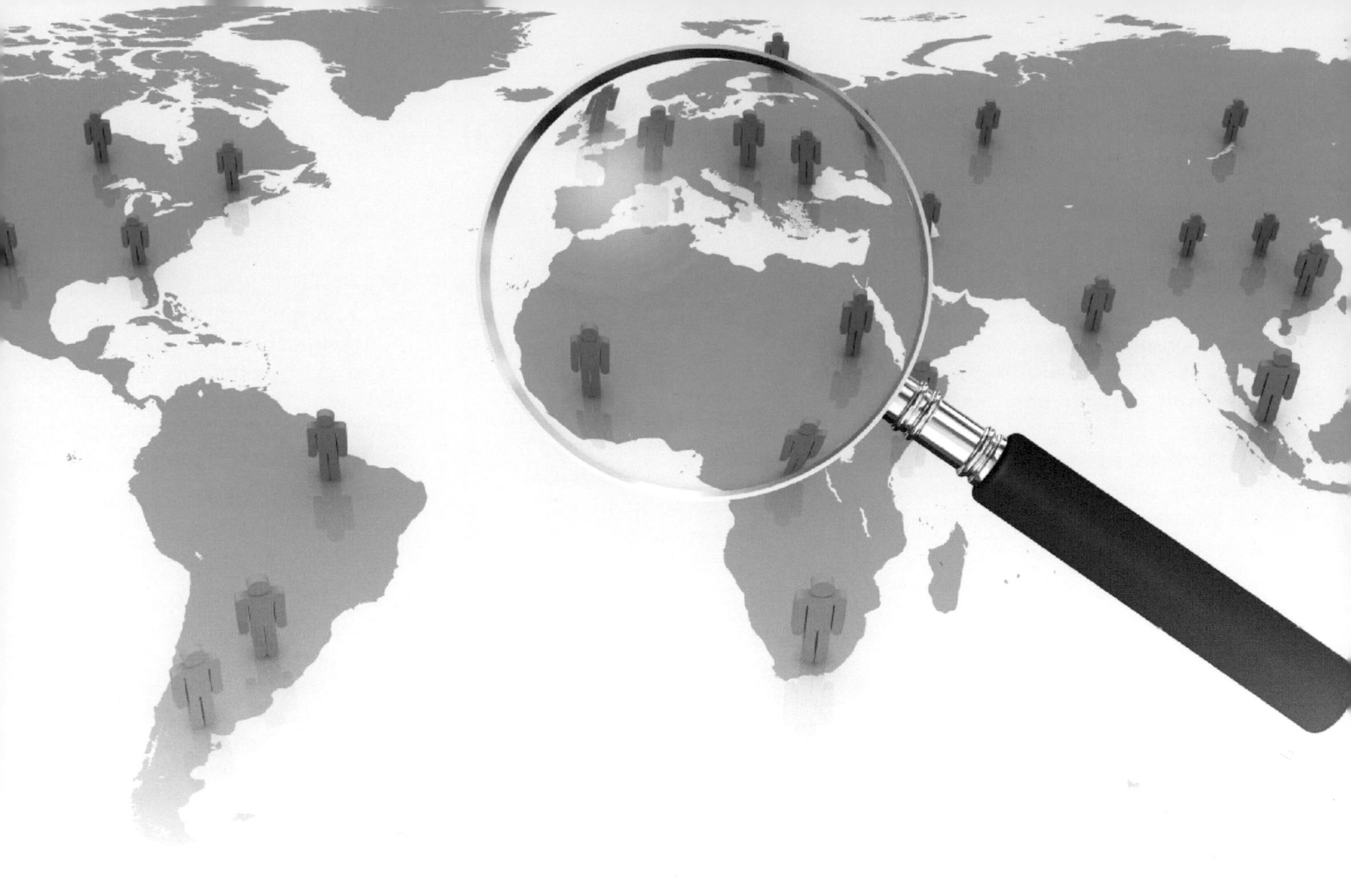

Healthcare systems around the world

A summary of healthcare systems in six different countries.

Australia

The current system is known as Medicare and supplements medical expenses for most healthcare required. Any remaining costs are paid for by the individual patient and those who earn above a certain income threshold are subject to an additional 1% tax if they choose to use the public system - encouraging many wealthier people to use private medical care.

Canada

A universal system that is mostly free. About 27% of Canadians' healthcare is paid for via private medical insurance, which covers things such as prescription drugs and dentistry.

France

A universal healthcare system in which the majority of medical expenses are paid for by the Government - usually 70% - and the rest can be claimed through supplemental medical insurance. Most long-term conditions entitle the patient to claim back 100% of their medical expenses.

Netherlands

Health insurance coverage is compulsory but is provided by private insurance companies.

Sweden

A reputation for low healthcare spending because of a system which encourages GPs to treat patients rather than refer them to specialists.

United States of America

Rated last in the quality of healthcare among similar countries by the Commonwealth Fund. Not all Americans are entitled to routine or basic healthcare services. Most people obtain medical insurance either through a private policy or through their employer. Others have to pay as-and-when they receive treatment.

12 August 2013

Let the NHS at 65 focus on safety and quality

One of Peter Cook's comic creations was a doddering grandee who had wasted years of his life trying to operate a restaurant serving only frogs and peaches, reflecting on whether he had learned from his mistakes. 'I think I have, yes, and I think I can probably repeat them almost perfectly,' he said.

The politicians in charge of the NHS not only repeat their mistakes, but define them rather differently than the rest of us.

Perhaps it all comes down to how you view the last 65 years. The vast majority of the public and professions see a service that has delivered remarkable outcomes for the money invested and that has somehow maintained founding principles of equity while the rest of society has become more unequal.

The politicians tend to see a service that has its moments, but is just one major reorganisation away from being perfect. The mistake, as they see it, is not to change the NHS more than they already have.

Previous anniversaries have been overshadowed by organisational change, but at 65 it is feeling akin to post-traumatic stress. And patients with this condition don't generally benefit from being repeatedly slapped around the face.

Instead of being allowed to emerge from the profound and deep trauma of the Health and Social Care Act, crises are being manufactured for political reasons. Conclusions are being manufactured before the evidence is gathered.

What has ever been achieved by the NHS being kicked around the parliamentary playground, other than demoralised staff and patients asking when the name-calling and meddling will stop?

But all is far from lost. Although many services are under enormous strain, they remain free at the point of delivery. This can and must remain the case. None of the alternatives would be better. Charging for NHS services would quite clearly bring back treatment based on the ability to pay. An insurance-based system brings with it an army of assessors trained to say 'no'. Means-tested charging would raise the spectre of minimalist state services for those who cannot afford private services. And there is little or no evidence that charging for services would reduce the share of national wealth spent on healthcare – and good evidence that it would reduce service access to an unacceptably low level for some groups.

Whatever is happening around us, it is important, as Nye Bevan did, to believe in a better future.

It is possible that those of us who are still working in the NHS in 10 years' time will speak of a service where healthcare professionals have been empowered to base their services on the best evidence, both clinical and structural, where the focus will be on quality and safety, and not on whichever organisational shape is in fashion, or the myth of the competitive market.

To get there, politicians have to end this obsession with NHS organisational form, each seeking to raze and rebuild their predecessor's work at enormous cost. Instead, they should talk to the patients, as we who work in the health service do every day, and to the staff. Listen to their voices and use them to improve services for everyone, rather than an excuse for further reorganisation. There are so many ways the NHS could be made better, without needing yet another New Jerusalem.

This article was written for *The Wisdom of the Crowd: 65 views of the NHS at 65*, published by the Nuffield Trust.

3 July 2013

⇨ The above information is reprinted with kind permission from the British Medical Association (BMA) and was originally published by Nuffield Trust. Please visit www.bma.org.uk or www.nuffieldtrust.org.uk for further information.

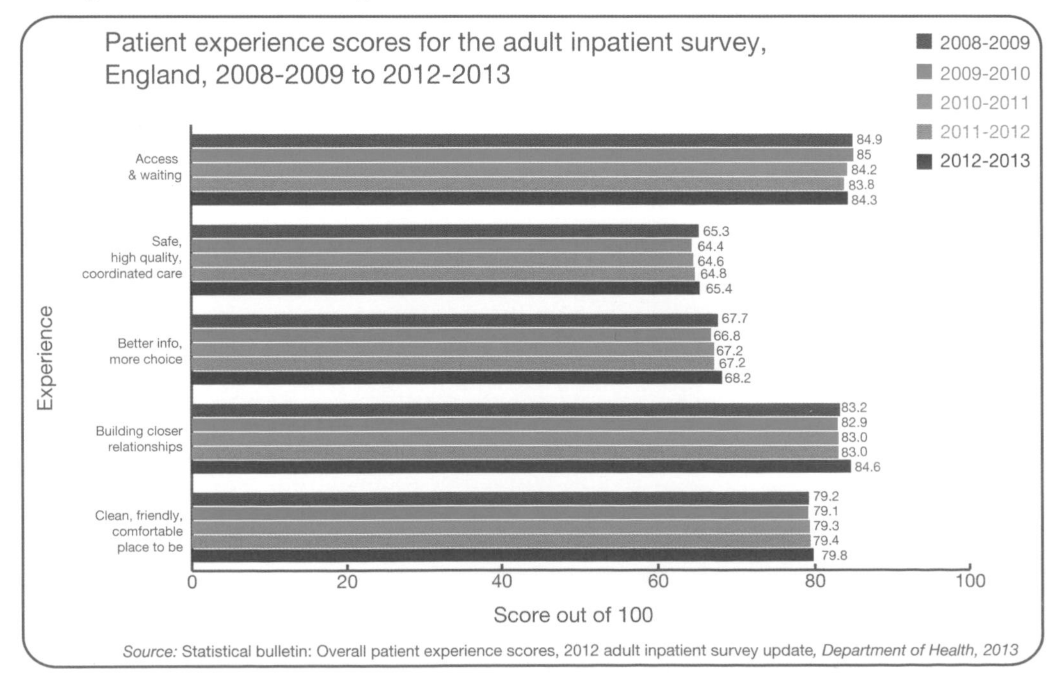

Patient experience scores for the adult inpatient survey, England, 2008-2009 to 2012-2013

Source: Statistical bulletin: Overall patient experience scores, 2012 adult inpatient survey update, *Department of Health, 2013*

Chapter 2

Healthcare problems

Elderly NHS patients left starving, thirsty and in pain, according to campaign charity report

Elderly patients in UK hospitals are being subjected to appalling standards of care, according to a report by the Patients Association.

The catalogue of abuse, highlighted in 16 cases, detail the neglect of the elderly, including cases where patients have been left starving or without pain relief.

The report also details cases whereby patients' families have been forced to care for their loved ones, as NHS staff were 'too busy'.

'Patients are being left sat in their own faeces and urine,' Angela Rippon, vice president of the Patients Association, told Sky News. 'It's unbelievable,' she added.

The dossier records the continuing decline in standards of care, despite Government promises that NHS hospitals would improve.

Health Secretary Andy Burnham said the report highlighted 'age discrimination' within the health service, while the head of the charity said it 'shamed everyone involved'.

Liz Kendall, Labour's Shadow Minister for Care and Older People, said the problems were partly due to pressures on the NHS, including 'increases in demand, squeezed resources and more very sick elderly patients ending up in hospital'.

'This report reveals yet more examples of vulnerable patients being denied basic standards of care that we would all expect for our elderly relatives. Such appalling treatment is unacceptable. NHS services that are falling short must be brought up to the standards of the best,' she added.

Cases highlighted in the report, include:

- Helena Grimwood, whose daughter claims that her mother was left 'desperately thirsty' as no one would help her take on fluids during her time at Southend University Hospital.
- Sally Abbott-Sienkiewicz who was left in 'horrendous' pain suffering from terminal cancer without pain relief when admitted to Glenfield Hospital in Leicester.
- William Wood who was admitted to hospital with swine flu. His wife told of how he pushed the emergency button because he was having trouble breathing but had to wait 15 minutes for assistance. Mr Wood collapsed and died following his release from York District Hospital.

Alongside the 16 cases, the Patients Association also recorded a 37% increase in the calls to its hotline in 2011.

'In the 21st century, in one of the most developed countries and health systems in the world, patients should not be left starving or thirsty, they shouldn't be left in pain and they shouldn't be left to defecate or urinate in their beds because the nurse designated to them says it's easier to change the sheets later than to help them to the toilet now,' said Katherine Murphy, chief executive of the Patients Association.

'These 16 are the tip of the iceberg. It's not always a problem of finance but a problem of attitude,' said Rippon.

'Nurses need university degrees, but you can't get a university degree in compassion.'

'This should not be happening.'

9 November 2011

- The above information is reprinted with kind permission from *The Huffington Post (UK)*. Please visit www.huffingtonpost.co.uk for further information.

Elderly patients' NHS care: your stories

There has been an outpouring of personal stories from* Guardian *readers following the Care Commission report on the poor treatment of elderly patients in NHS hospitals.

In October 2011, the Care Quality Commission released a report showing half of NHS hospitals are failing in their care of the elderly.

There's been an outpouring from *Guardian* readers of their personal stories of hospital treatment on the NHS.

Comments range from those who have direct experience of incredibly poor quality care ('on one visit she told us that she wanted to lie on the bed and die') – to those who countered these stories with experience of high-quality care ('I can't praise the healthcare professionals enough').

NHS workers have also explained their thoughts on the reasons behind the report.

'Ten years ago whilst incarcerated at the now defunct Ascot hospital in Berks, I witnessed first hand the lack of care for the elderly in many NHS hospitals.

'I was placed in a geriatric ward because there was no room in the general wards, many of the things I saw shocked me. I was left with a very reduced sense of respect for our health system.

'Toilets with no doors facing into a public area, patients having food placed in front of them and then removed later regardless of whether they had eaten or not, no help provided to old folk who could not feed themselves. One poor old dear had gone for two days with no food at all because of this regime before the rest of the "inmates" stepped in and started to feed her.

I would not like to be an elderly person in a British hospital if that is the standard of care.'

'We had two very different experiences of hospital care for the elderly with my mother, who recently died. She was initially admitted to a general hospital (Wycombe) with ovarian cancer (she also had dementia). The treatment both she and her relatives received was terrible, the doctors in particular were crass and insensitive. I was told by one Senior House Officer, whose second day it was on that particular ward, "we need our bed back so get her out of here".

'Luckily I managed, after a long fight, to get her transferred to a local cottage hospital where her care was wonderful. I cannot praise the staff (all staff) at Amersham enough. The care they provided for all the elderly people on the ward was second to none. Unfortunately, it is these very cottage hospitals that are under most threat. All the nurses there suggested that they might not have jobs in the very near future.

'Unfortunately, with Lansley's Bill being pushed through both Houses, I would suggest that our first experience of hospital care for the elderly would become the norm.'

'My mother was in a rather depressing ward. The nurses were kind enough, but the place was obviously understaffed. Cleanliness left a lot to be desired and the patients were rarely washed.

'One thing that got me was when I arrived to find my mother distressed and shivering because her blankets were on the floor. She asked a passing cleaner, a woman bringing drinks and the woman with the library trolley to replace them.

'They said that they were not allowed to because only nurses were allowed to touch bedding. Needless to say, it had been impossible to attract the attention of a nurse.'

'Two years ago my Grandmother was admitted to a Birmingham hospital at the age of 78 – immediately on arrival she was changed into a pair of incontinence pants despite the fact she was capable of going to the toilet if she had a little assistance in walking to the bathroom. The staff also tried to tell us that she had a great appetite and was eating very well... turns out she couldn't even swallow, so how she managed to eat all of these meals I'll never know!

She passed away after being in there for three days.

'A year later my grandfather was admitted to another Birmingham hospital known locally as "No Hope Hospital". He spent his first night on a trolley in A&E – he was there for 2 days before he passed away. I'm sad to say my heart sank when I found out they had been admitted to these hospitals, both of which have awful reputations – I just hope I don't have to get to that stage where I'm reliant on disinterested healthcare workers who just see me as a burden. I know there are lots of doctors and nurses out there who do their very best to provide excellent healthcare and to look after elderly patients, but sadly I just haven't experienced this yet.'

'My mum had worked as a nurse and always put patient care first and foremost. She always wanted to be a nurse and started nursing straight from school and rose through the ranks to be ward sister at a major London hospital.

'When she retired she approached a local hospital to volunteer on the wards at meal times. She was told that she could cut up food but must not under any circumstances feed patients, as if they choked this would be a health and safety issue. She offered to attend a course to "learn" how to feed a patient (despite the fact that she'd managed to do this for 20 years without incident!) but was told she was unable to.

'In the end she was so upset at seeing uneaten food being taken away from patients who were clearly unable to feed themselves and at the general level of patient care, something she said wouldn't have been allowed when she was nursing, that she stopped volunteering. When her husband was later admitted to hospital she ensured that she was there every meal time to feed him and help him wash and visit the toilet.'

'My experience as a previously registered manager of three care homes inspected by the Care Quality Commission is very positive but I know this depended on which area of the country you are in.'

'I've nursed in both the NHS and the private sector, and in my experience the standard of care in the private sector, especially private nursing homes, is much worse. A lot of private nursing homes save money by understaffing, refusing to buy enough supplies (pads, etc.), taking on low-paid poorly skilled nurses. These organisations refuse to deal with abuse or neglect by staff as it could harm their reputation if they do so, or in a lot of cases, owners just don't care as long as they're making money.

'To single out the NHS for this is missing the point entirely, although I suppose we'll get a lot more of these anti-NHS stories now the Bill's gone through – PR in advance for when the Government sign over hospitals to crappy private sector providers.'

'My grandma was admitted to an NHS hospital with a suspected stroke and was later moved when we discovered it was inoperable cancer. She had excellent care throughout and the nurses were superb and looked after her incredibly well.

'It's deeply worrying to hear the stories being reported but I think it's important to remember that this isn't everyone's experience. It seems there is a danger here of confusing bad practice at specific hospitals with a general malaise in the NHS.'

'Maybe I live in a parallel universe. I have just come out of hospital after a week in a ward populated by older people. The care could not have been better. Nurses, doctors and ancillary staff all went out of their way to ensure we were as comfortable as possible. Meals and snacks were offered on a regular basis. Nurses checked blood pressure, temperature etc. several times a day and ward assistants were always around. Beds were changed daily and I was checked every half hour because I could not walk and needed a "bottle".

'It seems very convenient that an anti-NHS report is issued just in the week the Tories want to demolish the NHS.'

13 October 2011

⇨ The above information is reprinted with kind permission from *The Guardian*. Please visit www.guardian.co.uk for further information.

Mid Staffordshire NHS Foundation Trust public inquiry

Letter to the Secretary of State, The Rt Hon Jeremy Hunt MP.

Dear Secretary of State,

Report of the Mid Staffordshire NHS Foundation Trust Public Inquiry

As you know, I was appointed by your predecessor to chair a public inquiry under the Inquiries Act 2005 into the serious failings at the Mid Staffordshire NHS Foundation Trust. Under the Terms of Reference of the Inquiry, I now submit to you the final report.

Building on the report of the first inquiry, the story it tells is first and foremost of appalling suffering of many patients. This was primarily caused by a serious failure on the part of a provider Trust Board. It did not listen sufficiently to its patients and staff or ensure the correction of deficiencies brought to the Trust's attention. Above all, it failed to tackle an insidious negative culture involving a tolerance of poor standards and a disengagement from managerial and leadership responsibilities. This failure was in part the consequence of allowing a focus on reaching national access targets, achieving financial balance and seeking foundation trust status to be at the cost of delivering acceptable standards of care.

The story would be bad enough if it ended there, but it did not. The NHS system includes many checks and balances which should have prevented serious systemic failure of this sort. There were and are a plethora of agencies, scrutiny groups, commissioners, regulators and professional bodies, all of whom might have been expected by patients and the public to detect and do something effective to remedy non-compliance with acceptable standards of care. For years that did not occur, and even after the start of the Healthcare Commission investigation, conducted because of the realisation that there was serious cause for concern, patients were, in my view, left at risk with inadequate intervention until after the completion of that investigation a year later. In short, a system which ought to have picked up and dealt with a deficiency of this scale failed in its primary duty to protect patients and maintain confidence in the healthcare system.

The report has identified numerous warning signs which cumulatively, or in some cases singly, could and should have alerted the system to the problems developing at the Trust. That they did not has a number of causes, among them:

- A culture focused on doing the system's business – not that of the patients;
- An institutional culture which ascribed more weight to positive information about the service than to information capable of implying cause for concern;
- Standards and methods of measuring compliance which did not focus on the effect of a service on patients;
- Too great a degree of tolerance of poor standards and of risk to patients;
- A failure of communication between the many agencies to share their knowledge of concerns;
- Assumptions that monitoring, performance management or intervention was the responsibility of someone else;
- A failure to tackle challenges to the building up of a positive culture, in nursing in particular but also within the medical profession;
- A failure to appreciate until recently the risk of disruptive loss of corporate memory and focus resulting from repeated, multi-level reorganisation.

I have made a great many recommendations, no single one of which is on its own the solution to the many concerns identified. The essential aims of what I have suggested are to:

- Foster a common culture share by all in the service of puttir the patient first;
- Develop a set of fundament standards, easily understoo and accepted by patients, th public and healthcare staff, th breach of which should not b tolerated;
- Provide professionally endorse and evidence-based mean of compliance with thes fundamental standards whicl can be understood and adoptec by the staff who have to provid the service;
- Ensure openness, transparenc and candour throughout the system about matters o concern;
- Ensure that the relentless focus of the healthcare regulator is on policing compliance with these standards;
- Make all those who provide care for patients – individuals and organisations – properly accountable for what they do and to ensure that the public is protected from those not fit to provide such a service;
- Provide for a proper degree of accountability for senior managers and leaders to place all with responsibility for protecting the interests of patients on a level playing field;
- Enhance the recruitment, education, training and support of all the key contributors to the provision of healthcare, but in particular those in nursing and leadership positions, to

integrate the essential shared values of the common culture into everything they do;

- Develop and share ever improving means of measuring and understanding the performance of individual professionals, teams, units and provider organisations for the patients, the public and all other stakeholders in the system.

In introducing the first report, I said that it should be patients – not numbers – which counted. That remains my view. The demands for financial control, corporate governance, commissioning and regulatory systems are understandable and in many cases necessary. But it is not the system itself which will ensure that the patient is put first day in and day out. Any system should be capable of caring and delivering an acceptable level of care to each patient treated, but this report shows that this cannot be assumed to be happening.

The extent of the failure of the system shown in this report suggests that a fundamental culture change is needed. This does not require a root and branch reorganisation – the system has had many of those - but it requires changes which can largely be implemented within the system that has now been created by the new reforms. I hope that the recommendations in this report can contribute to that end and put patients where they are entitled to be – the first and foremost consideration of the system and everyone who works in it.

Yours sincerely,

Robert Francis QC

Inquiry Chairman

5 February 2013

- The above information is an extract from the Mid Staffordshire NHS Foundation Trust Public Inquiry report. Please visit www.midstaffordshirepublicenquiry.com for further information.

Liverpool Care Pathway, controversial NHS end-of-life care, 'to be phased out'

An independent review of a controversial end-of-life regime is likely to recommend that it is phased out, it has emerged.

The review of the the Liverpool Care Pathway (LCP), chaired by crossbench peer Baroness Julia Neuberger, has been hearing evidence from patients, families and health professionals.

The LCP – which recommends that in some circumstances doctors withdraw treatment, food and water from sedated patients in their final days – has come under intense scrutiny.

Reports have suggested that doctors have been establishing 'death lists' of patients to be put on the pathway.

Articles have also claimed hospitals might be employing the method to cut costs and save bed spaces.

But medics have argued that the pathway has 'transformed' end-of-life care, saying it can offer peaceful, pain-free deaths when used properly.

A Department of Health spokeswoman said last night: 'The independent review into end-of-life care system the Liverpool Care Pathway, commissioned last year by Care and Support Minister Norman Lamb and backed by Health Secretary Jeremy Hunt, is likely to recommend that the LCP is phased out over the next six to 12 months.

'The review panel, set up by ministers following reports from families concerned about the care of their loved ones, is due to report back on Monday.

'It is expected to say that when used properly the LCP can give people a dignified and peaceful death, but that they found numerous examples of poor implementation and worrying standards in care which mean it needs to be replaced.'

Lamb told *The Daily Telegraph*: 'I took the decision to launch this review because concerns were raised with me about how patients were being cared for and how families were being treated during this difficult and sensitive time.

'We took those concerns very seriously and decided that we needed to establish the facts of what was happening so we could act where needed.'

He added: 'We need a new system of better end-of-life care tailored to the needs of individual patients and involving their families.'

British Medical Association president elect Baroness Finlay said the LCP was originally brought in because patients were 'dying badly, in hospitals in particular'.

They were being 'walked past, ignored and neglected', she said, and the LCP was an attempt to 'roll out the best of hospice care into other areas'.

'By and large that worked well but the problem has been that it hasn't always been used properly,' she told BBC Radio 4's *Today* Programme.

13 July 2013

- The above information is an extract from the article *Liverpool Care Pathway, controversial NHS end-of-life care 'to be phased out'* and is reprinted with kind permission from *The Huffington Post (UK)*. Please visit www.huffingtonpost.co.uk for further information.

The Francis Report: right diagnosis but will the treatment work?

By Stephen Thornton

'We have still not moved away from a culture of blame'. So says Robert Francis in his erudite, if voluminous, report into the failings at the Mid Staffordshire NHS Foundation Trust published earlier today.

He gets straight to the point in his report. The culture of the NHS still has too many negative aspects to it:

- a lack of openness to criticism
- a lack of consideration for patients
- defensiveness
- looking inwards not outwards
- secrecy
- misplaced assumptions about the judgements and actions of others
- an acceptance of poor standards
- and a failure to put the patient first in everything that is done.

All this must change, he quite rightly states.

He has some excellent ideas for how this can be achieved. Mercifully, he makes it clear he does not believe that structural change is the answer. He states it is unlikely that any structural change could enhance patient safety and goes on to make the telling point that within any system, of whatever design, there needs to be a relentless focus on ensuring patient safety.

The most welcome recommendation he makes is that the NHS Constitution should lie at the heart of the changes needed. 'The common values of the service must be enshrined in and effectively communicated by the NHS Constitution, and owned and lived by all members of the service', he states in the report. The Constitution should be the first reference point for all NHS patients and staff. As a member of the Expert Advisory Group on the NHS Constitution working with the Department of Health to modernise and promote a revised Constitution, this is music to my ears.

There are many other recommendations of real merit. For example, he rightly recognises the value of peer review, often neglected in a culture of top-down performance management. It has, he says, 'a far more fundamental role in changing behaviour to ensure a consistent and caring culture throughout healthcare services'.

He also helpfully recognises that there should be an increased focus on a culture of compassion and caring in nurse recruitment, training and education. He makes the valid point that training and continuous professional development for nurses should apply at all levels from student to director. We know how access to this is currently difficult, if not impossible, for many nurses. It will have resource implications but is vital to improve the quality of care.

It is gratifying too to see him recommend that the GMC and the NMC should ensure that patient safety should become the first priority of both medical and nursing training and education.

But as I waded through his report (the executive summary alone extends to 117 pages), I began to wonder: where is the patient in all this? I couldn't help but form an impression that the patient was there to be 'done unto'. In the case of Mid Staffordshire, done unto neglectfully and appallingly. In that context, Francis' quest was to find ways of ensuring that this would never happen again, that the patient in future would be put first, and everything done by the NHS and everyone associated with it should be informed by this ethos. Yet I could not help feeling that, in Francis' vision of the future, the patient remains something of a passive onlooker, not an assertive participant.

Quite properly, he says that, in the future, staff should put patients before themselves; they should do all in their power to protect patients from avoidable harm; and they should be open and honest with patients. Patients should be given information on which to make informed decisions. They, and the wider public, should be involved in decisions, both nationally and locally, about how care and treatment should be provided. Interestingly, specifically in relation to the care of elderly people, he also advocates a greater role for patients' families and carers.

However, nowhere does he say that patients should be involved in decisions about their care and treatment. Nowhere does he make it clear that it is the patients who should be in control. Nowhere does he advocate the encouragement of supported self-management. This is a missed opportunity to promote a step change in the way in which care is delivered in the NHS. It runs the risk of an undue reliance on the system getting it right for the patient. We know all too well that this is not enough.

6 February 2013

- The above information is reprinted with kind permission from The Health Foundation. Please visit www.health.org.uk for further information.

A&E waiting times reach nine-year high

Figures from the King's Fund show that nearly six per cent of patients waited for four hours or longer in accident and emergency in the final quarter of last year.

Waiting times for accident and emergency patients reach a nine-year high, according to latest figures.

The monitoring report from the King's Fund showed that in the final quarter of 2012/2013, 5.9 per cent of patients (313,000 people) waited for four hours or longer in A&E – the highest level since 2004.

This is an increase of more than a third on the previous three months, and of nearly 40 per cent since the same quarter the previous year.

It means that the Government's target that no more than five per cent of patients should wait for more than four hours has been broken for the first time since June 2011, when it pledged to keep waiting levels low.

Worrying

John Appleby, chief economist at the King's Fund, said: 'Emergency care acts as a barometer for the NHS. The worryingly high number of patients waiting longer than four hours in the last quarter of 2012/2013 is a clear warning sign that the health system is under severe strain.

'The pressures in emergency care will not be relieved by focusing on a single aspect of the problem in isolation– it requires a co-ordinated response across the whole health system.

'While the NHS is in a healthy financial position overall, efficiencies are becoming harder to deliver as one-off savings such as cuts in management costs start to slow. This is compounded by the need to maintain staffing levels following the shocking failures of care highlighted by the Francis Report.

'With staff costs making up the bulk of the NHS budget, this will leave little room for manoeuvre – significant changes to services will be required if the NHS is to meet its target of delivering £20 billion in efficiency savings.'

It follows a report that operations are regularly cancelled and led to an angry tweet from Shadow Health Secretary Andy Burnham.

Waiting times breached

Nearly 40 per cent of trusts reported that they breached the waiting time target in the last quarter. The King's Fund also said that the proportion of patients waiting more than four hours before being admitted to hospital from A&E has risen to nearly seven per cent – again, the highest level since 2004.

The charity said the analysis shows the 'severe strain on emergency care in early 2013' and that there is a risk the same thing could happen next winter.

However, a spokeswoman for the King's Fund said: 'Despite the pressures in emergency care, other NHS performance measures are continuing to hold up well. Waiting times for referral to treatment in hospital, the number of healthcare-acquired infections and delays in transferring patients out of hospital all remain stable.'

A survey of NHS finance directors also conducted by the King's Fund found that the NHS is set to end the 2012/2013 period in a healthy financial position, but that the outlook for the following two years is bleak.

4 June 2013

⇨ The above information is reprinted with kind permission from Channel 4. Please visit www.channel4.com/news for further information.

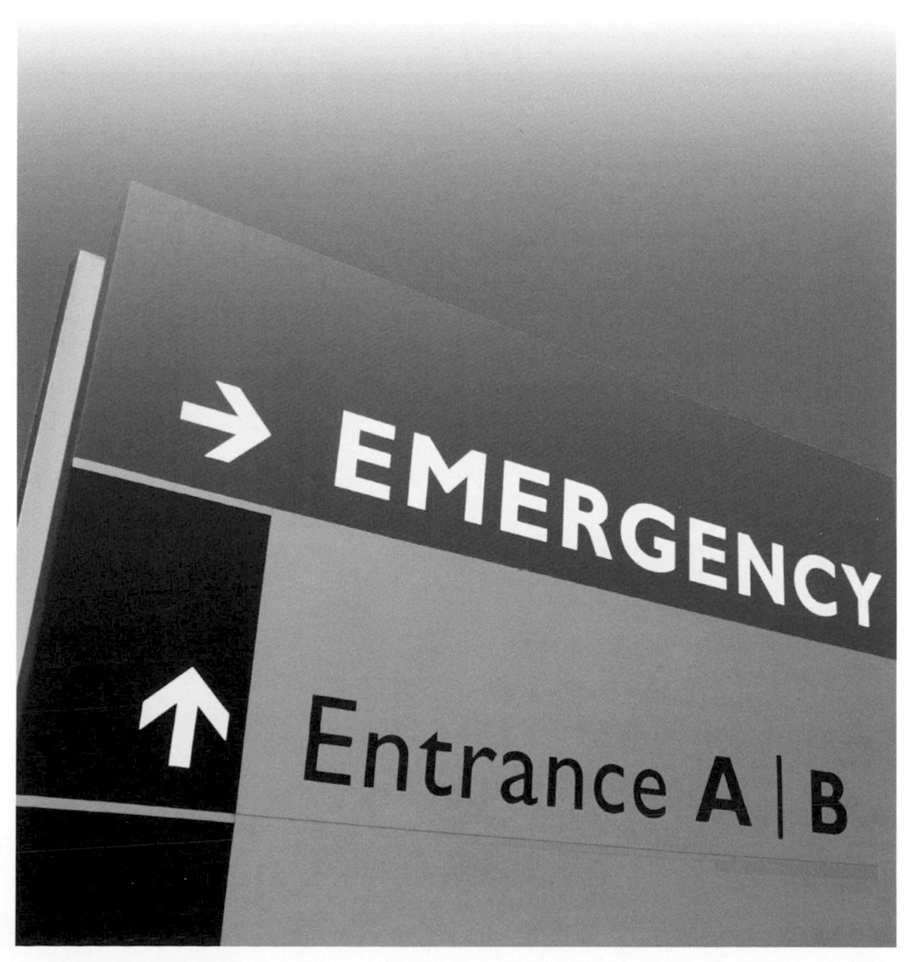

Statistical press notice: the 2012 NHS Staff Survey in England

Key points from the latest release include:

- 63 per cent of NHS staff said that if a friend or relative needed treatment they would be happy with the standard of care provided by their organisation. This figure is unchanged from that in the 2011 survey. In addition, 62% said that care of patients and service users is their organisation's top priority.
- There continues to be an improvement in the proportion of staff receiving appraisals, up from 80% in the 2011 survey to 83% in 2012, however, only 36% of staff said these appraisals were well structured.
- Only 40% of all staff were satisfied with the extent to which they felt that their trust values their work – this figure is lowest for ambulance staff (23%) and highest amongst social enterprise staff (47%). However, the proportion of staff who indicated that they would recommend their organisation as a place to work has increased for the first time in three years (55% in 2012 compared to 51% in 2011, 53% in 2010 and 55% in 2009).
- Only 35% said that communication between senior managers and staff is effective, this figure is the lowest for ambulance staff (20%), and less than a third of all NHS staff (26%) reported that senior managers act on feedback from staff. Despite this, 74% said that they are able to make suggestions on how they could improve the work of their team or department.
- 15 per cent of NHS staff reported experiencing physical violence from patients, their relatives or other members of the public in the previous 12 months and 30% of all staff report that they experienced bullying, harassment and abuse from patients, their relatives or other members of the public in the previous 12 months. Just under two-thirds of incidents of physical violence and 44% of bullying, harassment and abuse cases were reported. The questions relating to such experiences were changed for the 2012 survey and so comparisons with earlier surveys are not appropriate.

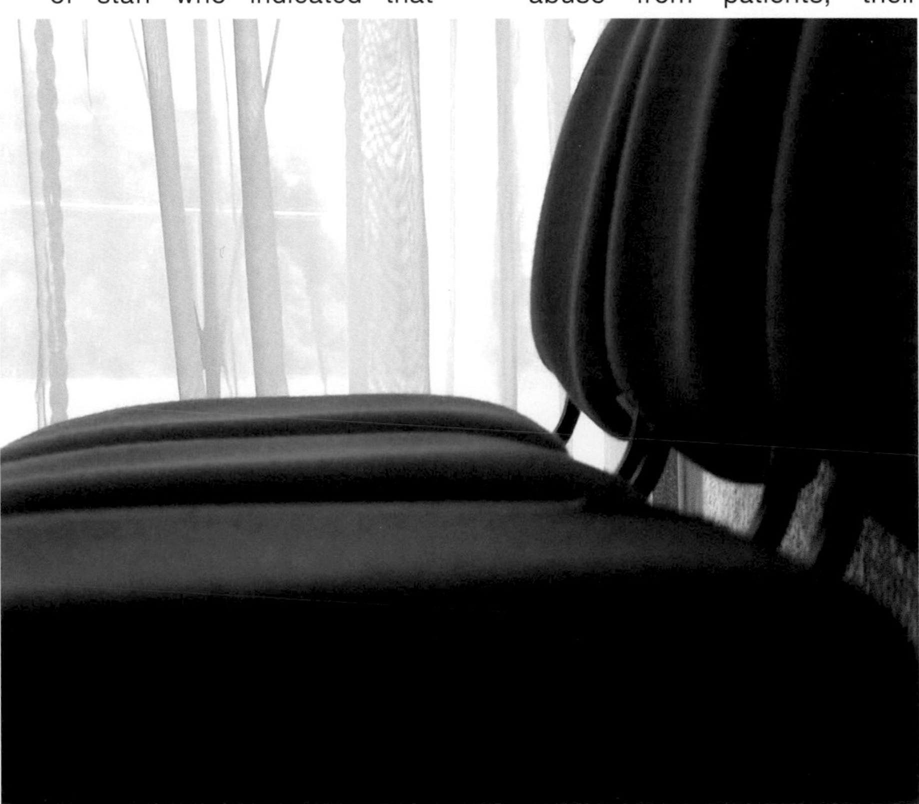

Notes on the survey

The 2012 NHS Staff Survey covered 259 NHS organisations in England. 203,000 NHS staff were invited to participate using a self-completion postal questionnaire survey method. 101,169 responses were received – a response rate of 50% (compared with 54% in 2011). All full-time and part-time staff who were directly employed by an NHS organisation on 1 September 2012 were eligible. Commissioning PCTs were given the option not to participate in the survey; four Commissioning PCTs chose to participate. Fieldwork for the survey was carried out between late September and early December 2012. The results are weighted so that they reflect unbiased estimates of all NHS staff in England. Because of changes made to improve and shorten the survey for 2012, a number of the key findings are not directly comparable with their equivalents in previous years.

28 February 2013

- The above information is reprinted with kind permission from the Department of Health. Please visit www.gov.uk for further information.

Healthcare in Britain: is there a problem and what needs to change?

Healthcare in Britain – and the National Health Service (NHS) in particular – has been affected by significant shifts in the policy and economic landscapes in recent years. In 2011-2012, as the country grappled with the economic standstill and the Coalition Government's austerity policies started to bite, the NHS began the year with virtually no increase in real funding. After a decade when real spending doubled, the NHS has been allocated little extra funding over and above inflation until April 2015, with the prospect of a continuing freeze for some years beyond that. The productivity task that the NHS has been set in response to this squeeze on its finances is unprecedented. By 2015, a virtually unchanged NHS budget will have to generate an extra 20 per cent more value – the equivalent of around £20 billion of extra funding for the NHS in England alone. Given that there has been little or no improvement in productivity during the past decade and a half, this represents a huge challenge.

The timing of the latest British Social Attitudes survey was also significant in wider policy terms as interviews took place when the Government was pursuing its controversial Health and Social Care Bill through Parliament. Now an Act of Parliament (2012), this provides for what the Chief Executive of the NHS in England has memorably described as reforms so big 'they could be seen from space'. At the heart of the changes lies the abolition of Primary Care Trusts and the transfer of the budgets and responsibility for commissioning most NHS services to local clinical commissioning groups (CCGs) led by general practitioners (GPs).

The challenges in terms of both increasing productivity and reforming services rest on an understanding that the NHS is experiencing a 'problem' that needs 'fixing'. Regarding the former, the problem is fairly easy to perceive: how to maintain a quality service with virtually zero real growth in funding and growing needs. However, regarding reform – while acknowledging that performance and organisation in healthcare can always be improved to some degree – the problem has been less easy to identify. A central criticism of the Coalition's reform plans for the English NHS has been not just that they lack a persuasive narrative about the need for change, but also that they lack evidence that change is necessary on the scale proposed. Indeed, the previous British Social Attitudes survey carried out in 2010 seemed to provide evidence to the contrary by showing that 70 per cent of people were satisfied with the way the NHS runs – the highest level recorded since the survey began in 1983 (Clery, 2011).

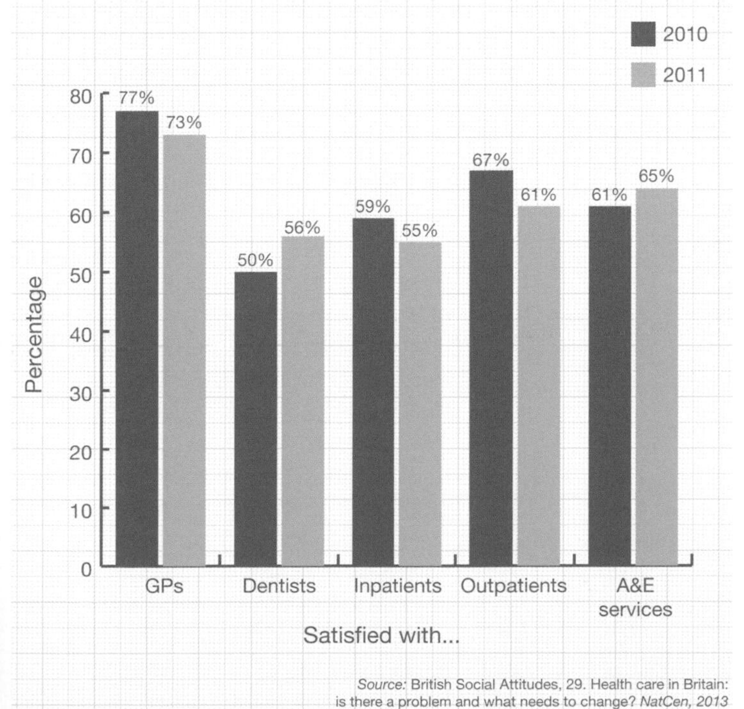

Source: British Social Attitudes, 29. Health care in Britain: is there a problem and what needs to change? *NatCen, 2013*

How, in the context of an impassioned debate about the future of the NHS, have public attitudes towards the NHS changed since then? This article firstly explores the public's views about how the NHS is performing, looking at satisfaction with services and perceptions of change over recent years, and seeks to explain why opinion has shifted. Secondly, in the light of the wider debate about whether the fundamental nature of the NHS will – or should – change in response to the intensifying pressure on funding, the article looks to the future, exploring public attitudes to radical changes in the way the NHS is funded and accessed as well as its priorities for spending.

Does the NHS need to change and, if so, how?

Overall satisfaction with the NHS, although it remains quite high, has taken a sharp downturn since 2010. The proportion of the population who think the service has improved over the last five years has also declined. But what are respondents' thoughts on the future of the NHS?

For the first time, the latest survey asked people if they thought the general standard of healthcare in the NHS would improve or get worse in the next five years. In line with our thesis that current dissatisfaction relates to the level of public uncertainty about NHS reform, more than a third believe that NHS healthcare will get worse. They outnumber the roughly one in four who consider it will improve.

This pessimistic view chimes with a Department of Health survey of NHS staff, which showed that 53 per cent of those surveyed in the winter of 2011 felt the standard of NHS care to patients would get worse – an increase over the result of the winter 2010 survey (49 per cent) and the spring 2009 survey (34 per cent).

We then looked at what enthusiasm, if any, exists for changing the NHS by asking:

In general, would you say that the healthcare system in Britain needs no changes, needs a few changes, needs many changes, or, needs to be completely changed?

The replies suggest an appetite for modest, though possibly not radical, reform. Over half (55 per cent) believe that 'a few changes' are needed, and another third (32 per cent) that the NHS requires 'many changes'. Only five per cent say that no change is necessary – which is also the proportion who maintain that the service 'needs to be changed completely'. Since this question has not been asked in previous British Social Attitudes surveys we cannot assess how the public's view may have changed over time. Nevertheless, having established that most people favour at least some reform of the NHS, we move on to consider what types of change they are most likely to support.

Tax, public spending and the future of the NHS

Those who feel Britain's health system needs to be improved are faced with a number of choices as to how to do this. Three fundamental ones are what public spending priority to assign to health; what the scope of health services should be; and who should have access to them. We start by examining what spending priority the public assigns to health versus other areas of government spending, and people's personal willingness to pay more to improve healthcare. We also test people's confidence that a National Health Service funded through general taxation will remain the chosen model for providing healthcare in the future. Since people generally favour reform, might not some believe that it is the NHS's founding ambition to provide a comprehensive, universal healthcare service that most needs to change?

Support for more taxation to pay for public services has been on the decline since 2002. Having stood at 63 per cent ten years ago it has now fallen to 36 per cent in the latest survey (though this is up five percentage points from 2010). Correspondingly, there has been an increase in the proportion saying the Government should 'keep taxes and spending at the same level', from 31 per cent in 2002 to 54 per cent in the latest survey – a trend in part reflecting increases in spending in some key areas (such as the NHS) over this period: as more is spent, a decreasing proportion of the public see the need to spend even more.

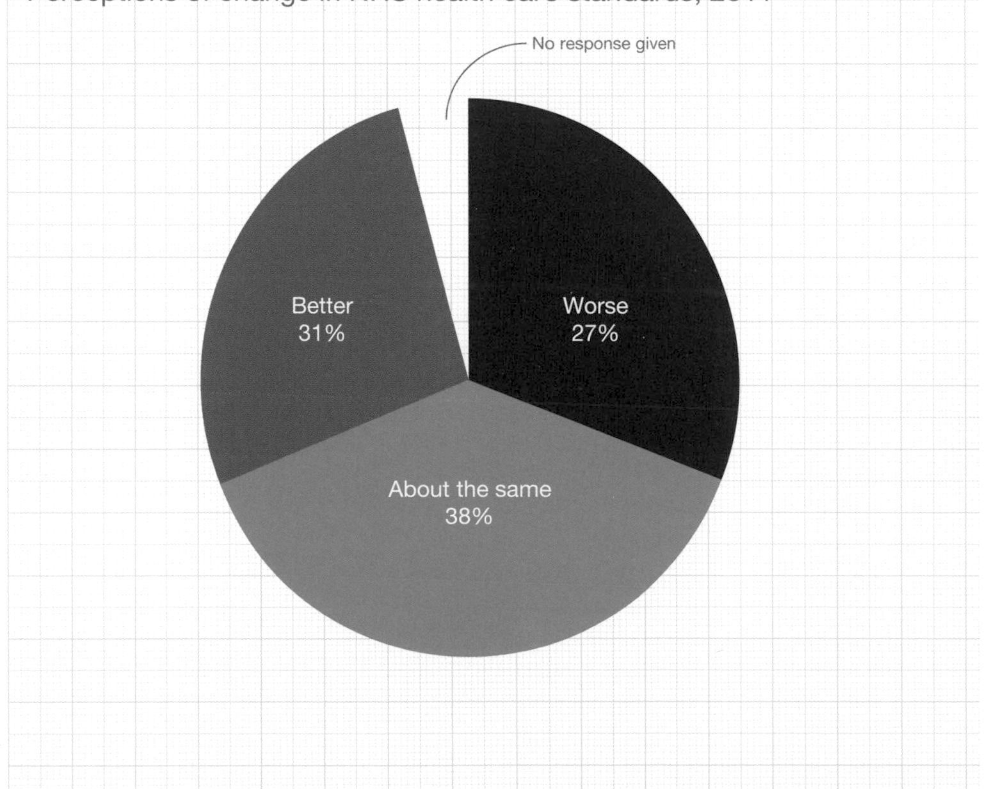

Source: British Social Attitudes, 29. Health care in Britain: is there a problem and what needs to change? *NatCen, 2013*

British Social Attitudes also asks people to choose from a list one area of Government spending they would prioritise for extra spending, and then to select an area as their second choice. When first and second choices are added together, health has consistently been the public's top priority, with 68 per cent choosing health in the current survey. Education comes a reliable second, while other areas of government spending such as police and prisons and housing (the third and fourth top priorities in 2011) are given much lower priority. The priority that the public accords to health can, in a sense, be said to accord with the Coalition Government's spending priorities, which are to hold level the amount of money going to the NHS, while other areas undergo extensive cuts. However, it is interesting to note the general decline in the priority given by the public to the NHS for extra funding since the turn of the century. As with the declining proportion of those who want higher taxes and more spending on public services in general, this is a trend that perhaps mirrors the funding increases the NHS has received since that time; as more money goes in, the public have perceived less need for increased funding. Of interest too is the fact that this decline in the priority accorded to the NHS continues in 2011. This might suggest that worries about funding are not in fact a significant factor explaining the fall in satisfaction with the NHS.

Our next question investigates people's own willingness to pay higher taxes in order to improve the level of healthcare 'for all people in Britain'. In line with opinions on the question of whether taxation should rise to fund public services, we find that nearly four in 10 (38 per cent) say they would be prepared to pay more. Another one in four (26 per cent) say they would be neither willing nor unwilling, while almost one in three (31 per cent) would be unwilling. We find a significant link (at the 90 per cent level) between satisfaction with the NHS and willingness to pay more to support the service. So it could be that steps to ease funding constraints would be a way to arrest the current decline in public satisfaction.

When we compare the answers to this and the previous question by demographic group, we find those who favour raising taxes to pay for public spending in general are outnumbered in most groups by those who would be willing to pay more tax to fund the NHS in particular. Willingness to pay more tax to fund the NHS is especially strong among people aged 55 to 64, among Labour and Liberal Democrat supporters, and among those with higher academic qualifications. Conservative supporters, although least likely to give a positive answer to either question, are noticeably more likely to express willingness to pay more tax themselves to benefit the NHS than to support tax increases for public services in general.

An alternative to 'tax and spend' could be to reduce the scope of what the NHS offers by limiting access. For example, we ask:

It has been suggested that the National Health Service should be available only to those with lower incomes. This would mean that contributions and taxes could be lower and most people would then take out medical insurance or pay for healthcare. Do you support or oppose this idea?

The answers show that, for more than 20 years now, the proportion opposing this suggestion 'a lot' or 'a little' has consistently remained at or above 70 per cent. (The lowest level of opposition – and the highest level of support – was recorded back in 1983 when the then Prime Minister, Margaret Thatcher, was at her most popular.) The latest survey does, however, show a dip in opposition and an increase in support for a healthcare system based on medical insurance or direct payment. But the proportion in favour of changing the NHS funding model is still below 30 per cent.

In a similar vein, but without referring to income, the latest British Social Attitudes survey also asks how much people agree or disagree that 'the Government should provide only limited healthcare services'. Again, 73 per cent voice opposition to the proposition. However, the level of agreement is much lower than for the previous question at just nine per cent.

Percentage of people willing to pay more tax for increased health spending to improve healthcare

Age group	Percentage
18-34	35%
35-54	35%
55-64	47%
65+	41%

Source: British Social Attitudes, 29. Health care in Britain: is there a problem and what needs to change? *NatCen, 2013*

We also ask what people believe will happen in reality:

In ten years' time, do you think the NHS will still be paid for by taxes and free to all?

The public is not overwhelmingly confident that the service's traditional funding model will survive. While just under half (47 per cent) reply 'yes', a very similar proportion (44 per cent) say 'no'. When we look at this against people's reported levels of satisfaction with the NHS overall we see that those who think the NHS will not be free and available to all in ten years' time are significantly less likely to express satisfaction with the service now (50 per cent, compared with 63 per cent of those who think the NHS will remain freely accessible). Whether a view that the NHS will not be tax-funded and free to all in future causes lower satisfaction now or vice versa is impossible to say. Furthermore, it cannot be assumed that everyone who thinks NHS funding and access will change in future necessarily regards this is a bad thing – although the responses to our previous question on limiting access to the NHS do suggest that most would see this as a negative change.

While many feel the NHS needs to change to some degree, radical changes to its funding source and the scope of its services are not generally the kind of change they have in mind. Even so, a large minority think this is what will, in fact, happen.

Setting priorities and commissioning local health services

While the Coalition Government's reforms stop short of any fundamental changes to the NHS as a publicly-funded, universal and comprehensive service, the administrative changes it is implementing are nevertheless far-reaching. As previously noted, the key reform is the creation of local clinical commissioning groups run by GPs, replacing primary care trusts as the purchasers of secondary care. The central argument advanced for this change has been that GPs are better placed to make decisions about priorities and spending as they are closer to patients. But who do the public think can best decide how NHS money is spent? What sort of service priorities do they think the NHS should pursue and – more broadly – what kind of public health measures do they favour for promoting healthier living?

We asked people who they think 'should decide how money is spent on your local NHS' and offered them four options: 'the Government', 'your local GPs', 'your local council' and 'local people'. The responses show that there is no majority view. Around one in three say the spending decisions should be taken by local GPs, while just under a third consider that they should be the remit of central Government, and around one in six choose 'local people' or the 'local council' respectively. Broadly then, there is some support – though not overwhelming – for the central plank of the Government's reform programme to put GPs in charge of deciding how around 60 per cent of the NHS budget should be spent.

Regardless of who makes the decisions about healthcare spending, any NHS service commissioner faces difficult choices about the priorities for that spending. To test public opinion about the types of health spending that should receive priority, given limited resources, we invited respondents to imagine they had charge of an NHS budget, with 40 'beans' or counters to allocate between four specific areas of spending. These were selected broadly to represent community services ('increase community nurses to support people with long-term health problems in their own homes'), hospital care ('reduce hospital waiting times for people who need a hip operation'), mental health treatment ('expand access to counselling and "talking therapies" for mild/moderate depression') and preventive public health services ('give more help for people who need to lose weight').

Aggregating the way people allocated their beans across these four areas produces the distribution shown in. We see that respondents collectively earmark 38 per cent of the hypothetical health budget for community nursing services. Public support for this sort of service, helping people with long-term conditions at home, chimes with professional efforts over many years to shift care provision towards the community where appropriate, rather than providing it in hospitals. The strength of support for more investment in community services may also reflect a feeling that, notwithstanding the long term shift in policy, such care continues to be underfunded. It is also interesting that despite substantial reductions in the waiting times for operations and other hospital treatments in recent years, the public votes to allocate as much as 30 per cent of its notional health budget to reduce the time that people need to wait for a hip operation.

Support for the mental health option is given less priority, attracting 20 per cent of the notional budget, while the lowest share (12 per cent) is given to support for public health through a weight loss programme. The low priority given to this last choice may, in part, reflect a feeling among some people that helping people who need to lose weight is not even an appropriate activity for the NHS: looking at the way individuals allocate their budget beans we find that as many as three out of ten respondents allocated none of them to the public health option.

Ways to improve public health

To investigate further what kinds of public health intervention people consider more or less acceptable, we asked them to say what in their view would be 'the best way for the Government to help people to lead healthier lifestyles'. The options they chose between were:

- ⇨ Leave people to make their own choices without interfering
- ⇨ Provide information (e.g. on healthy diets, how to give up smoking)
- ⇨ Pay people (e.g. to give up smoking or take more exercise)
- ⇨ Use the law (e.g. to ban drinking in public places)
- ⇨ Tax unhealthy things (e.g. alcohol and cigarettes).

In general, the public is less keen on what might be termed 'hard' interventions – such as using the law (nine per cent) or paying people in return for healthier behaviour (two per cent). The 'softer' approach that almost half say they favour is providing information on healthy diets. Despite the long standing practice of governments in taxing alcohol and tobacco for avowedly 'health' as well as 'revenue' reasons, we also see that little more than one in five think it offers the best way to promote healthier lifestyles. Just under one in five, meanwhile, take a libertarian view, insisting that people should be left to make their own health choices without Government interference.

2012

- ⇨ The above information is reprinted with kind permission from NatCen. Please visit www.bsa-29.natcen.ac.uk for further information.

Priorities for NHS spending

Respondentss felt that:

- **Increasing the number of community nurses to support people with long-term health problems in their own homes should receive 38% of the (hypothetical) budget.**
- **Reducing hospital waiting times for people who need a hip operation should receive 30% of the (hypothetical) budget.**
- **Expanding access to counselling and 'talking therapies' for mild/moderate depression should receive 20% of the (hypothetical) budget.**
- **Giving more help to people who need to lose weight should receive 12% of the (hypothetical) budget.**

Source: British Social Attitudes, 29. Health care in Britain: is there a problem and what needs to change? *NatCen, 2013*

Foreigners are taking advantage of the NHS, David Cameron says

Foreigners are taking advantage of the NHS and should only get free treatment if they have been paying taxes, David Cameron has said.

By Rowena Mason

The Prime Minister said Britain is 'not tough enough right now' about stopping health tourists coming to Britain to use the NHS.

Speaking to workers at B&Q in Eastleigh, Mr Cameron said the health service should not be free for foreigners from outside the EU. Britain must also get better at charging other EU countries when their citizens use the NHS, he added.

'We're not tough enough right now about people coming from the other side of the world who decide to use our health service,' he said. 'They haven't contributed in their taxes. They should pay when they use the NHS.'

Mr Cameron criticised the current system as he was asked about the pressure on NHS services if a wave of Bulgarians and Romanians immigrate to Britain when restrictions are lifted next year.

'We've made some progress but there's a lot more to do to make sure that while we're welcoming to immigrants we don't allow people to come here and take advantage of us, because I think that does happen too often,' he said.

Mr Cameron this week launched a review into how foreigners access benefits. On a visit to support the Conservative Eastleigh by-election campaign, he said this review will look at all welfare payments and services, including health, housing and legal aid as well as traditional benefits.

It comes after GPs wrote to ministers last month demanding changes to stop widespread health tourism costing the NHS millions of pounds a year.

Recent guidance states that immigration status should be no bar to being registered with a doctor. GPs point out that once a foreign patient has registered, hospital staff hardly ever check whether they are also entitled to more specialist NHS care.

A recent survey carried out by *Pulse* magazine has found 52 per cent of GPs thought NHS entitlements for migrants were too generous, while only seven per cent thought they were too stringent.

New guidelines from the Primary Care Commission state: 'Nationality is not relevant in giving people entitlement to register as NHS patients for primary care services.'

The guidelines also emphasise that anyone in the UK can register at a GP practice, no matter how long they have been in the country.

In 2010 a Department of Health report conceded that health tourism was costing the NHS at least £10 million a year in unrecovered costs, although doctors believe the true figure is far higher because most goes undetected.

14 February 2013

⇨ The above information is reprinted with kind permission from *The Daily Telegraph*. Please visit www.telegraph.co.uk for further information.

ER... ARE YOU A UK TAXPAYER?
HEY I PAID SOME TAX AT THE AIRPORT...
NHS

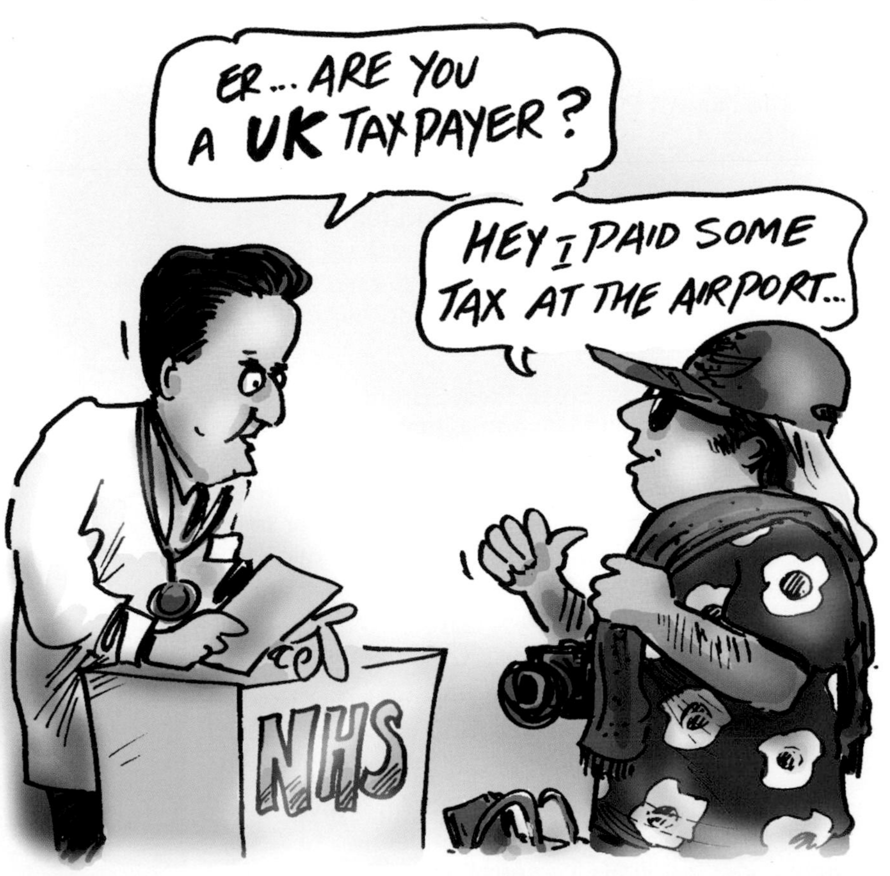

Immigrant family denied treatment on NHS for Erb's palsy baby Sanika Ahmed

By Felicity Morse

A baby denied NHS treatment because of her parents' immigration status may end up paralysed if she is not seen by doctors soon, her parents have said.

Sanika Ahmed was born in Hampshire to Bangladeshi parents but because their visa has expired, the Royal National Orthopaedic Hospital in Middlesex has refused her treatment.

The eight-month-old suffers from Erb's palsy and unless she has nerve graft surgery before she is nine months old, it is unlikely she will ever regain movement in her arm.

The hospital say that although Sanika is UK-born she is dependent upon her parents and therefore is not entitled to free NHS treatment. Her parents have already applied for permission to stay in the UK.

Sanika's mother, Syeda Ahmed, told the BBC that consultants have told her Sanika only has a month in which to be treated before she is permanently paralysed in her arm.

'Sanika is slowly, slowly getting paralysed and it is very upsetting for all our family,' she said.

Her father Muhammad Ahmed is from Bangladesh and though he had a legal permit to work in the UK from July 2008 to August 2009, he stayed on illegally after his permit ended.

Mr and Mrs Ahmed are attending an appeal hearing next month that will rule on their legal right to remain in the UK. The hospital has said it has offered to treat Sanika privately. The cost for such treatment is estimated to run into tens of thousands of pounds and her parents have said they cannot afford it.

Karen Hillyer from the Erb's Palsy Group told *The Huffington Post UK*: 'Most consultants would not operate after nine-ten months for nerve graft surgery because the results would be so disappointing. There's a variety of ancillary surgeries you can have after this point but nothing that would restore nerve function in the arm. You are looking at ameliorating the situation rather than restoring movement.'

The Royal National Orthopaedic Hospital said in a statement 'Sanika Ahmed was first referred to the Royal National Orthopaedic Hospital NHS Trust in July 2012 and again in October 2012.

'We contacted Sanika's parents on 8 November 2012 asking for standard proof of entitlement to NHS treatment under the NHS Overseas Patient Regulations.

'Mr and Mrs Ahmed's entitlement to live in the UK expired in August 2009. Although Sanika is UK-born she is dependent upon her parents and under the provisions of the NHS Overseas Patient Regulations, Sanika was not entitled to free NHS treatment.

'In February 2013 we received a letter from Mr Ahmed's legal representatives regarding this matter and we replied offering to treat Sanika as a private patient. We received no reply to this offer.

'We understand that Mr and Mrs Ahmed are attending an appeal hearing next month that will rule on their legal right to remain in the UK. We are happy to see Sanika as an outpatient pending the results of this appeal.'

13 March 2013

⇨ The above information is reprinted with kind permission from *The Huffington Post (UK)*. Please visit www.huffingtonpost.co.uk for further information.

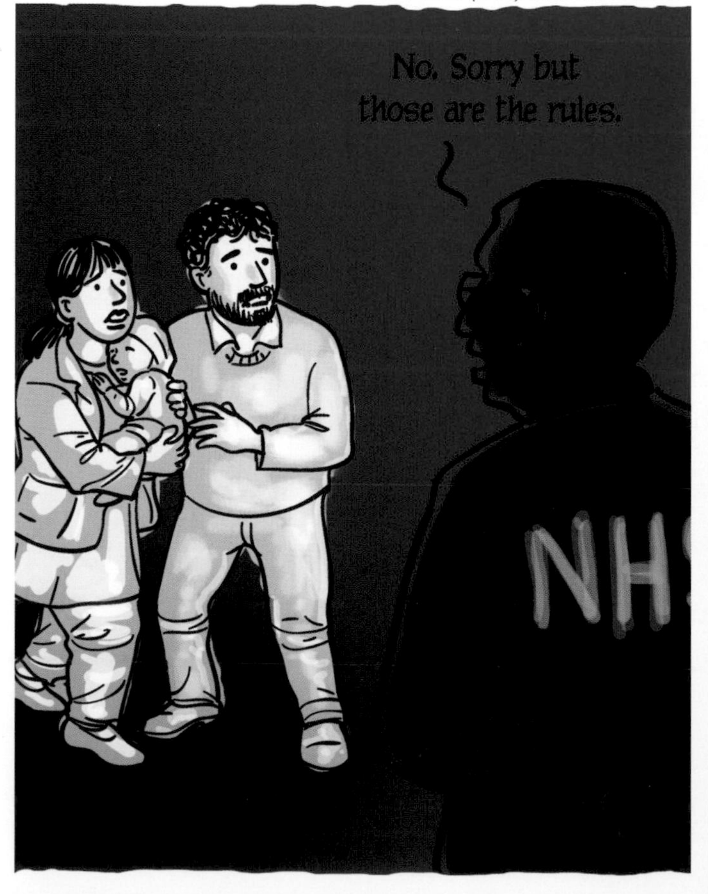

Chapter 3

The future of the NHS

Health and Social Care Act 2012

The Health and Social Care Act legislates for the reform of health and social care services in England. Passed in 2012, the Act introduces major changes to the way health and social care services are funded, commissioned and administered.

This article gives a brief guide to the new structure of services. It also explains the organisations that will regulate and monitor healthcare services, and details the main changes that patients will encounter.

The new structure of health and social care in England

The new structure of the health and social care services in England will be in place from April 2013. This will include new funding and commissioning bodies and new responsibilities for local authorities. Some of the main changes to key governmental agencies are outlined below:

The core values of public health services in England will change to include:

- The Secretary of State no longer has a duty to provide health services through the NHS, which increases the opportunity for private healthcare firms to deliver many services that were previously operated by the NHS.
- The Secretary of State does remain responsible for the NHS, setting objectives and retaining powers to intervene in emergencies through the Department of Health.
- The Secretary of State continues to set an overall budget for the NHS.
- Public health services must remain cost free to patients, except where other legislation specifically allows.

Strategic Health Authorities (SHAs), which manage local health services on behalf of the Department of Health, will be abolished and replaced by:

- A new National Commissioning Board (NCB), set up to provide leadership for local Clinical Commissioning Groups (see below) and commission some specialist and primary care services, such as GPs, dentists, community pharmacies and opticians. As well as a national office, the NCB will have a network of local area offices.
- A new body called Public Health England, created to provide leadership for local authorities (councils) in their new public health role and work with other bodies on promoting public health issues.

Primary Care Trusts (PCTs), which commission local primary care services and control around 80% of the NHS budget, will be abolished and replaced by:

- Clinical Commissioning Groups (CCGs): new GP-led bodies that are responsible for commissioning most health services, including primary care services such as GPs, dentists and pharmacies, and secondary care services such as those provided by hospitals. While CCGs will be led by GPs, the exact size and make-up of each group may be decided locally. Other professionals, such as nurses, practice managers, finance officers, council officials and representatives from the charity sector, may be part of a CCG.
- Local authorities (councils): Councils will take on the role of public health promotion, being responsible for measures to tackle issues such as obesity, smoking, health screening and vaccinations. councils will be required to consider health in all of their policies, for instance their existing duties towards social care, transport, housing and education. Each local authority will undertake a Joint Strategic Needs Assessment (JSNA) before April 2013, which defines local needs and priorities to be considered by the local Health and Well-being Board. CCGs are required to be mindful of these priorities when commissioning services.

Regulating and monitoring health and social care services

Some new bodies have been set up to monitor health and social care services in England, while the remit of other bodies has been extended to provide an extra level of regulation.

- The National Commissioning Board (NCB) described above is responsible for the regulation of GPs, including those who are members of CCGs.
- Monitor will regulate CCGs, community services and secondary care services. It will have a remit to protect and promote patients' interests, tackling abuses and unjustifiable restrictions of competition.

Essentially, it will act as an economic regulator for health and social care services in England, ensuring that NHS and private providers are able to compete fairly to run many services.

- The National Institute for Health and Clinical Excellence (NICE) will have its remit expanded to include the development of quality standards for social care. NICE will provide guidance to GPs, CCGs, community services and secondary care services.
- The Care Quality Commission (CQC) is responsible for ensuring that providers of health and adult social care services, such as the NHS, meet its standards of quality and safety. The CQC will regulate GPs, community services and secondary care services.
- Healthwatch is a new, independent service which aims to protect the interests of all those who use health and social care services. Healthwatch will have a role in communicating the views of patients to commissioning bodies and regulators and will be able to provide information, advice and support to members of the public. It will also have a say in the commissioning of services. Healthwatch England is the national body that governs a network of local Healthwatch organisations across the country. Further information and a directory of local services are available on the Healthwatch website.
- Health and Well-being Boards will bring together health and social care commissioners, councillors and lay representatives to promote joint working and tackle inequalities in people's health and well-being in their local area. From April 2013, Health and Well-being Boards will take over responsibility for refreshing the local JSNA, and developing a health and well-being strategy to promote public health issues across health, social care and other local services. Each local Healthwatch will have a seat on the boards, as will charity sector representatives in some cases. Health and Well-being Boards will also provide support to CCGs.

NCBs, the CQC and NICE are directly accountable to the Department of Health, which is in turn accountable to Parliament. Monitor is directly accountable to Parliament.

The complaints process

For members of the public who wish the make a complaint about health and social care services, the Patient Advice and Liaison Service (PALS) and the Independent Complaints Advocacy Service (ICAS) will remain. However, the local Healthwatch organisation will also be available from April 2013 to give advice and guidance to patients who are unhappy with the treatment they receive.

Complaints about health services will be referred to the appropriate NHS trust, GP or commissioner, with the Parliamentary and Health Services Ombudsman available if a local resolution cannot be reached.

Complaints about social care services are made to the relevant adult social services department, with the Local Government Ombudsman available if a local resolution cannot be reached.

The patient's perspective

The new NHS will give patients a choice over the services they choose. They will be able to register with a GP of their choice, regardless of where they live. When a patient is referred (usually by their GP) for a particular health service, they should be able to choose from a list of qualified providers who meet NHS quality requirements and price.

In theory, the new free-market system will reduce the number of targets on services from central government, and force them to focus on providing quality care to patients. Moving commissioning to the GP-led CCGs aims to ensure services are based on local needs and priorities. Patients may find that private companies are commissioned to deliver some services that were previously provided by the NHS or local authority.

Healthwatch will be an important contact for patients who would like to express their views on health and social care services. It aims to make it easier for commissioners to identify the needs of local people, and for patients to make their voices heard.

Acknowledgements

Headway would like to thank Somerset Link for their support in writing this guide.

- The above information is reprinted with kind permission from Headway – the brain injury association. Please visit www.headway.org.uk for further information.

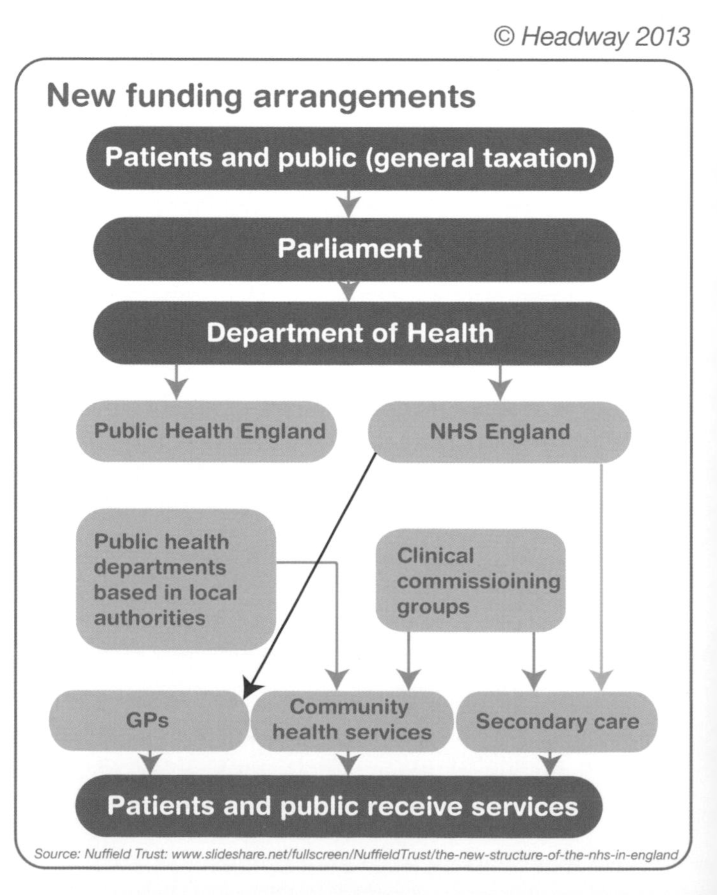

A mandate from the Government to the NHS Commissioning Board

The Mandate to the NHS Commissioning Board sets out the objectives for the NHS and highlights the areas of health and care where the Government expects to see improvements.

The Mandate focuses on the areas that matter most to people:

⇨ helping people live longer

⇨ managing ongoing physical and mental health conditions

⇨ helping people recover from episodes of ill health or following injury

⇨ making sure people experience better care

⇨ providing safe care.

Introduction

'The NHS belongs to the people. It is there to improve our health and well-being, supporting us to keep mentally and physically well, to get better when we are ill, and when we cannot fully recover, to stay as well as we can to the end of our lives. It works at the limits of science – bringing the highest levels of human knowledge and skill to save lives and improve health. It touches our lives at times of most basic human need, when care and compassion matter most. The NHS is founded on a set of common principles and values that bind together the communities and people it serves – patients and the public – and the staff who work for it.'

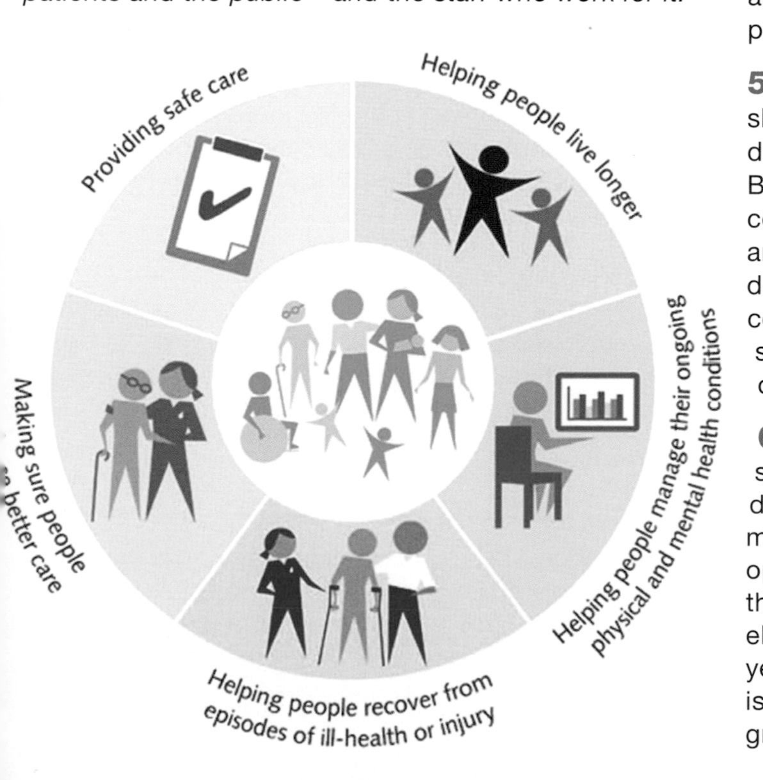

The NHS Constitution

1. As a nation, we are proud of what the NHS has achieved and the values it stands for. But public expectations of good healthcare do not stand still. So on behalf of the people of England, patients and those who care for them, this first mandate to the NHS Commissioning Board sets out our ambitions for how the NHS needs to improve. It covers the period from April 2013 to the end of March 2015.

2. It is the Government's privilege to serve as guardian of the NHS and its founding values. We will safeguard, uphold and promote the NHS Constitution; and this is also required of the NHS Commissioning Board.

3. The NHS is there for everyone, irrespective of background. The Government will continue to promote the NHS as a comprehensive and universal service, free at the point of delivery and available to all based on clinical need, not ability to pay. We will increase health spending in real terms in each year of this Parliament. We will not introduce new patient charges.

4. The creation of an independent NHS Commissioning Board, and this mandate to the Board from the Government, mark a new model of leadership for the NHS in England, in which ministers are more transparent about their objectives while giving local healthcare professionals independence over how to meet them.

5. The NHS budget is entrusted to the Board, which shares with the Secretary of State for Health the legal duty to promote a comprehensive health service. The Board oversees the delivery of NHS services, including continuous improvement of the quality of treatment and care, through healthcare professionals making decisions about services based on the needs of their communities. The Board is subject to a wide range of statutory duties, and is accountable to the Secretary of State and the public for how well it performs these.

6. This mandate plays a vital role in setting out the strategic direction for the Board and ensuring it is democratically accountable. It is the main basis of ministerial instruction to the NHS, which must be operationally independent and clinically-led. Other than in exceptional circumstances, including a general election, it cannot be changed in the course of the year without the agreement of the Board. The mandate is therefore intended to provide the NHS with much greater stability to plan ahead.

7. The Board is legally required to pursue the objectives in this document.[1] However it will only succeed through releasing the energy, ideas and enthusiasm of frontline staff and organisations. The importance of this principle is reflected in the legal duties on the Secretary of State and the NHS Commissioning Board as to promoting the autonomy of local clinical commissioners and others.

8. The scale of what we ask will take many years to achieve, but if the Board is successful, by March 2015 improvement across the NHS will be clear. By then, patients will see real and positive change in how they use health services, and how different organisations work together to support them.

9. The Government's ambition for excellent care is not just for those services or groups of patients mentioned in this document, but for everyone regardless of income, location, age, gender, ethnicity or any other characteristic. Yet across these groups there are still too many long standing and unjustifiable inequalities in access to services, in the quality of care, and in health outcomes for patients. The NHS is a universal service for the people of England, and the NHS Commissioning Board is under specific legal duties in relation to tackling health inequalities and advancing equality. The Government will hold the Board to account for how well it discharges these duties.

10. The objectives in this mandate focus on those areas identified as being of greatest importance to people. They include transforming how well the NHS performs by:

- preventing ill-health, and providing better early diagnosis and treatment of conditions such as cancer and heart disease, so that more of us can enjoy the prospect of a long and healthy old age;
- managing ongoing physical and mental health conditions such as dementia, diabetes and depression – so that we, our families and our carers can experience a better quality of life; and so that care feels much more joined up, right across GP surgeries, district nurses and midwives, care homes and hospitals;
- helping us recover from episodes of ill health such as stroke or following injury;
- making sure we experience better care, not just better treatment, so that we can expect to be treated with compassion, dignity and respect;
- providing safe care – so that we are treated in a clean and safe environment and have a lower risk of the NHS giving us infections, blood clots or bed sores.

11. These areas correspond to the five parts of the NHS Outcomes Framework, which will be used to measure progress. The framework will be kept up to date to reflect changing public and professional priorities, and balanced to reduce distortion or perverse incentives from focusing inappropriately on some areas at the expense of others. In order to allow space for local innovation at the front line, both the Government and the NHS Commissioning Board will seek to ensure that local NHS organisations are held to account through outcome rather than process objectives. As one of its objectives, the Board will need to demonstrate progress against the five parts and all of the outcome indicators in the framework – including, where possible, by comparing our services and outcomes with the best in the world.

12. As part of this, the Government has identified the following priority areas where it is expecting particular progress to be made: (i) improving standards of care and not just treatment, especially for older people and at the end of people's lives; (ii) the diagnosis, treatment and care of people with dementia; (iii) supporting people with multiple long-term physical and mental health conditions, particularly by embracing opportunities created by technology, and delivering a service that values mental and physical health equally; (iv) preventing premature deaths from the biggest killers; (v) furthering economic growth, including supporting people with health conditions to remain in or find work. The Board is also expected to play a full role in supporting public service reform.

13. These priorities reflect the Government's absolute commitment to high-quality healthcare for all, while highlighting the important additional role the NHS can play in supporting economic recovery.

14. The Mandate is not exhaustive. As part of the changes in the relationship between the Government and the NHS, the Board has agreed to play its full part in fulfilling pre-existing government commitments not specifically mentioned in the Mandate. For its part, the Government will exercise discipline by not seeking to introduce new objectives for the Board between one mandate and the next.

15. In all it does, whether in the Mandate or not, whether supporting local commissioners or commissioning services itself, the Commissioning Board is legally bound to pursue the goal of continuous improvement in the quality of health services.

13 November 2012

- The above information is an extract from the report *A mandate from the Government to the NHS Commissioning Board: April 2013 to March 2015.* Please visit www.gov.uk for further information.

1 See section 13A(2) of the National Health Service Act 2006, as inserted by the Health and Social Care Act 2012

The NHS is not ready for reforms, experts warn

Health experts have issued a stark warning that the NHS is 'not ready' on the day that massive changes in the organisation come into effect.

The Health and Social Care Act, which became law after a tortuous passage through Parliament, is expected to cost the taxpayer between £1.5 billion and £1.6 billion to implement.

Nick Black, professor of health service research at the London School of Hygiene and Tropical Medicine, said that he did not believe the health service was prepared for such a huge structural change.

He warned that hospitals could 'grind to a halt' as cuts to social care budgets mean that doctors are unable to discharge patients who do not need to be on the wards.

When asked whether the NHS is ready for such a big change, Black said: 'Not really no. It could really do without this.

'What we have got at the moment is a perfect storm with three major things happening – the changes in the structure, the fall out from Francis and the Nicholson challenge (where the NHS has been tasked with making £20 billion in efficiency savings during the four years to 2015).

'At one level patients won't notice anything dramatic on Monday morning.

'But the biggest thing that patients will notice will be the knock-on effect from the cuts in social care funding. It is clear that our hospitals are already struggling to discharge patients.

'Hospitals could cease to function and the system could grind to a halt because of people who do not need to be there.'

Rachael Maskell, head of health at union Unite, added: 'There is every indication that the NHS is not ready for the changes. The time scale was totally unrealistic.'

Labour said that the reforms have exposed the health service to risk because they have been implemented during a time of huge financial pressure.

The main aim of the health reforms was to make the NHS more accountable to patients and to release frontline staff from excessive bureaucracy and top-down control.

One of the biggest changes is the move from primary care trusts (PCTs) to clinical commissioning groups (CCGs), which will be led by GPs and other clinicians who will take on responsibility for commissioning care. The move will see 211 CCGs replace 151 PCTs across England.

But last week it was announced that only half of the new CCGs will be fully ready to start work when the changes come into effect on April 1. Just 106 CCGs are 'fully authorised', said NHS England.

The Department of Health said that for the first time health and social care services will be 'designed around the needs of the local community'.

A spokesman said that under the new system patients will be given more choice in who provides their care and a stronger voice through a new consumer champion Healthwatch England and the 'friends and family test'.

Health Minister Lord Howe said: 'The NHS needs to change so that patients get the care they need, when they need it.'

He added: 'Health and care services will be better joined up by bringing together the NHS, local councils and patients.

'Patients will have a greater influence in changes to their local health and care services through the patient-led inspections and the friends and family test.'

1 April 2013

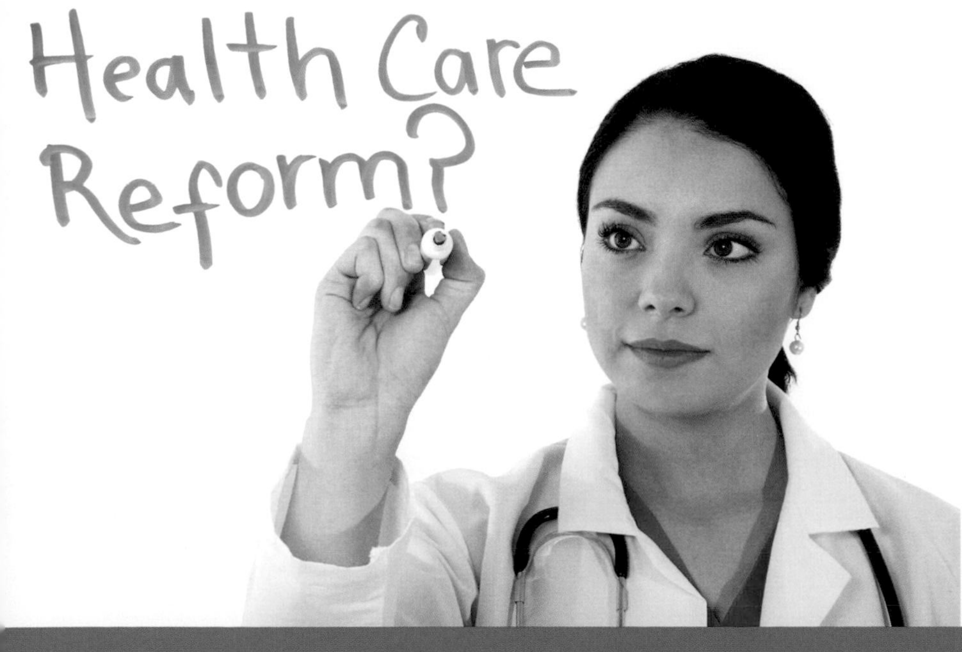

⇨ The above information is reprinted with kind permission from *The Huffington Post UK*. Please visit www.huffingtonpost.co.uk for further information.

The NHS structure explained

The NHS is undergoing major changes in its core structure. Most of the changes took effect on 1 April 2013, though some were in place before then. It will be some time before all the changes are fully implemented. All vital NHS services will continue as usual during the transition period and beyond.

These changes will have an effect on who makes decisions about NHS services, how these services are commissioned, and the way money is spent.

Some organisations such as primary care trusts (PCTs) and strategic health authorities (SHAs) will be abolished, and other new organisations such as clinical commissioning groups (CCGs) will take their place.

NHS services will be opened up to competition from providers that meet NHS standards on price, quality and safety, with a new regulator (Monitor) and an expectation that the vast majority of hospitals and other NHS trusts will become foundation trusts by 2014.

In addition, local authorities will take on a bigger role, assuming responsibility for budgets for public health. Health and well-being boards will have duties to encourage integrated working between commissioners of services across health, social care, public health and children's services, involving democratically elected representatives of local people. Local authorities are expected to work more closely with other health and ca providers, community groups and agencies, using th knowledge of local communities to tackle challeng such as smoking, alcohol and drug misuse and obesi

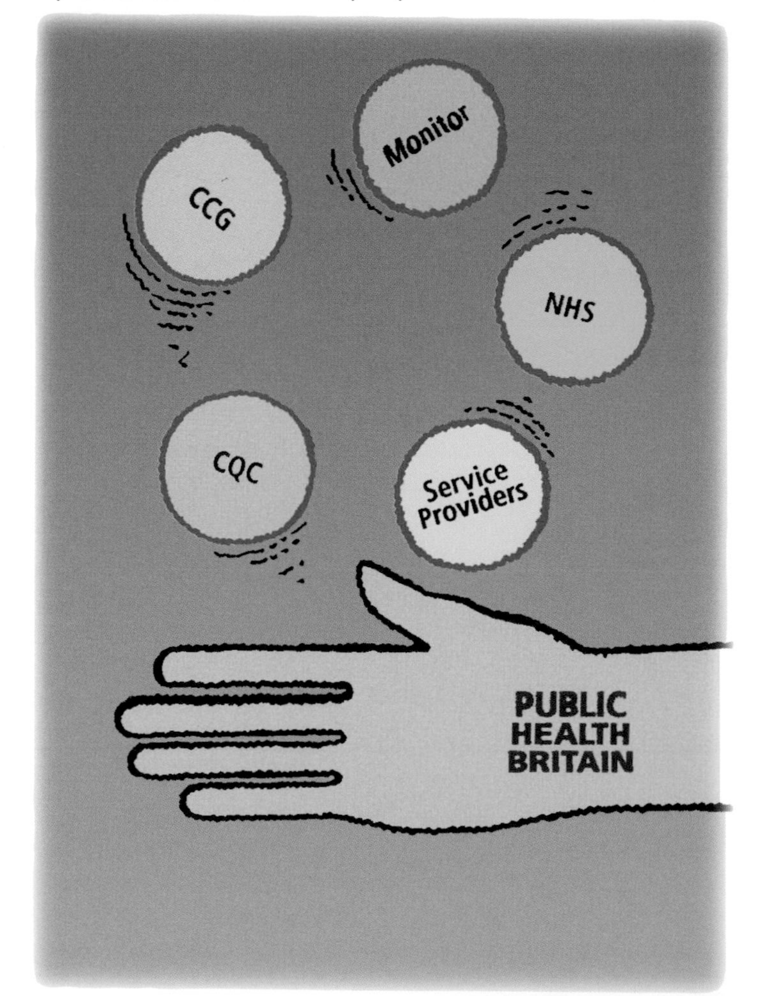

However, none of these changes will affect how y access NHS services in England. The way you book yc GP appointment, get a prescription, or are referred a specialist will not change. Healthcare will remain fr at the point of use, funded from taxation, and based need and not the ability to pay.

Overview of organisations and their role

The Secretary of State for Health

The Secretary of State for Health has ultima responsibility for the provision of a comprehensive hea service in England and ensuring the whole system wor together to respond to the priorities of communities a meet the needs of patients.

The Department of Health

The Department of Health (DH) will be responsible strategic leadership of both the health and social ca systems, but will no longer be the headquarters of t NHS, nor will it directly manage any NHS organisatior For detailed information about the department's n priorities and roles visit the DH website.

NHS England

Formerly established as the NHS Commissioning Boa in October 2012, NHS England is an independent bo at arm's length to the Government. Its main role is improve health outcomes for people in England. It wil

- provide national leadership for improving outcom and driving up the quality of care
- oversee the operation of clinical commissioni groups
- allocate resources to clinical commissioning grou
- commission primary care and specialist services.

For more information, visit NHS England.

Clinical commissioning groups (CCGs)

Primary care trusts (PCTs) used to commission m NHS services and controlled 80% of the NHS budg On April 1 2013, PCTs were abolished and replac with clinical commissioning groups (CCGs). CCGs have taken on many of the functions of PCTs and in addition some functions previously undertaken by the Department of Health.

All GP practices belong now to a CCG and the groups also include other health professionals, such as nurses. CCGs commission most services, including:

- ⇨ planned hospital care
- ⇨ rehabilitative care
- ⇨ urgent and emergency care (including out-of-hours)
- ⇨ most community health services
- ⇨ mental health and learning disability services.

CCGs can commission any service provider that meets NHS standards and costs. These can be NHS hospitals, social enterprises, charities or private sector providers.

However, they must be assured of the quality of services they commission, taking into account both National Institute for Health and Care Excellence (NICE) guidelines and the Care Quality Commission's (CQC) data about service providers.

Both NHS England and CCGs have a duty to involve their patients, carers and the public in decisions about the services they commission.

The health and care system from April 2013

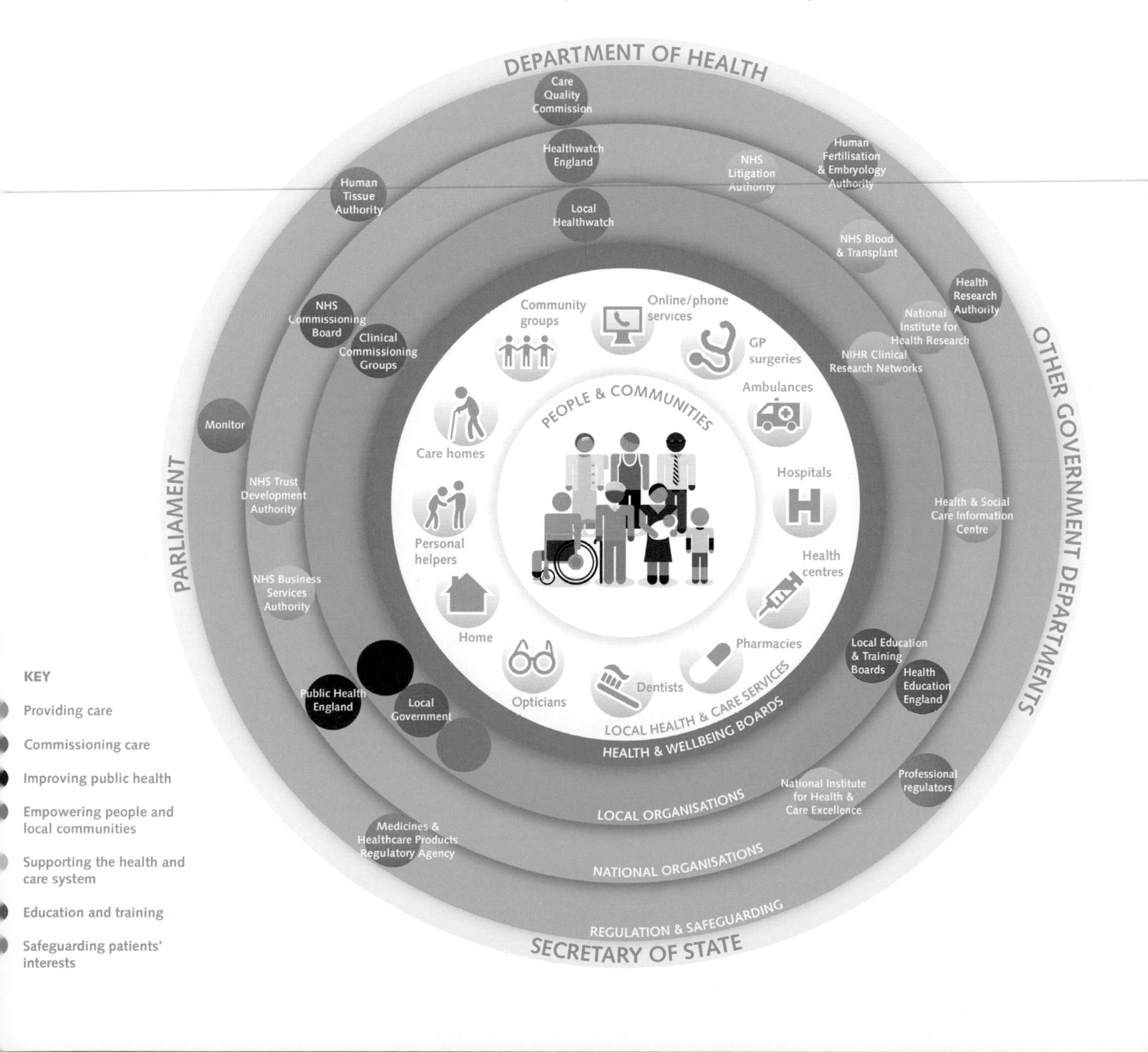

Health and well-being boards

Every 'upper tier' local authority is establishing a health and well-being board to act as a forum for local commissioners across the NHS, social care, public health and other services. The boards are intended to:

- ⇨ increase democratic input into strategic decisions about health and well-being services
- ⇨ strengthen working relationships between health and social care
- ⇨ encourage integrated commissioning of health and social care services.

Public Health England

A new organisation is also being created; Public Health England (PHE) will provide national leadership and expert services to support public health and will also work with local government and the NHS to respond to emergencies. PHE will:

- ⇨ coordinate a national public health service and deliver some elements of this
- ⇨ build an evidence base to support local public health services
- ⇨ support the public to make healthier choices
- ⇨ provide leadership to the public health delivery system
- ⇨ support the development of the public health workforce.

'NHS services will be opened up to competition from providers that meet NHS standards on price, quality and safety'

Regulation – safeguarding people's interests

Since April 2013, some elements of the regulation system have changed. Responsibility for regulating particular aspects of care is shared across a number of different bodies, such as:

- ⇨ the Care Quality Commission
- ⇨ Monitor
- ⇨ individual professional regulatory bodies, such as the General Medical Council, Nursing and Midwifery Council, General Dental Council and the Health and Care Professions Council
- ⇨ other regulatory, audit and inspection bodies – some of which are related to healthcare and some specific to the NHS.

The Care Quality Commission (CQC)

The CQC continues to regulate all health and adult social care services in England, including those provided by the NHS, local authorities, private companies and voluntary organisations.

Monitor

Monitor expanded its role to regulate all providers of health and adult social care services. Monitor aims to promote competition, regulate prices and ensure the continuity of services for NHS foundation trusts.

Under the new system, most NHS providers will need to be registered with both the CQC and Monitor to be able to legally provide services.

Note: all service providers are required to hold a licence issued jointly by the CQC and Monitor. To get a licence, providers will need to meet essential standards of quality and safety. They'll also have to follow certain behaviours relating to price setting, integrated care and competition. More importantly, providers will have to ensure services don't stop in the event of financial difficulties. If a provider does not fulfil the terms and conditions of the licence, both Monitor and CQC can take independent action, such as issuing warning notices or financial penalties.

Healthwatch

Healthwatch is a new organisation and functions as an independent consumer champion, gathering and representing the views of the public about health and social care services in England.

It operates both at a national and local level and ensures the views of the public and people who use services are taken into account.

Locally, Healthwatch will give patients and communities a voice in decisions that affect them, reporting their views, experiences and concerns to Healthwatch England. Healthwatch England will work as part of the CQC.

Other changes to the regulation system

- ⇨ Following the abolition of strategic health authorities (SHAs), the NHS Trust Development Authority (NHS TDA) will be responsible for overseeing the performance, management and governance of NHS Trusts, including clinical quality, and also managing their progress towards foundation trust status. The TDA has a range of powers, from appointing chairs and non-executive directors, to requiring a trust to seek external advice.

28 January 2013

- ⇨ The above information is reprinted with kind permission from NHS Choices. Please visit www.nhs.uk for further information.

Will the Friends and Family Test improve quality in the NHS?

By Chris Graham

There's a tendency in the NHS to be ruthlessly target-driven. Often, it goes like this: a scandal or a public outcry leads ministers to demand improvement, a 'magic bullet' metric is identified, and providers are made accountable for delivering against targets. Examples are plentiful, as are perverse incentives and unintended outcomes. Take the 48-hour target for GP access: incentivising GPs to provide a high proportion of appointments within two working days simply prompted the withdrawal of advance bookings. Cue jammed phone lines, the practice on auto redial at 8.30am, call back tomorrow or come in and hope for a gap. A target comprehensively hit at the expense of patient care.

If outcry continues to drive a target culture, it is inevitable that the tragedy of Mid Staffordshire will cast a long shadow over what and how we seek to improve. Certainly the Inquiry has already influenced political language: Jeremy Hunt speaking of a 'crisis of care' in some parts of the NHS, Robert Francis himself, during the Inquiry, talking of 'a tsunami of anger' threatening to 'overwhelm' those who fail to engage with and listen to patients and the public. Measuring, understanding and improving the experience of patients is now, and will remain, absolutely centre stage.

The NHS has long been ahead of the curve in measuring experience. It gathers a wealth of qualitative and quantitative information from a wide range of sources, and has had a suite of gold-standard national survey programmes in place for a decade.

The Friends and Family Test represents data collection on a whole new scale. From 1 April 2013, all hospitals in England will be expected to give every discharged adult inpatient or A&E attendee the opportunity to complete the Friends and Family Test. Given a target response rate of 15-20%, this is close to four million responses a year. The key requirement is for one question: 'How likely are you to recommend our ward/A&E department to friends and family if they needed similar care or treatment?'. Responses to this question will be collated nationally and acute trusts will be paid under CQUIN arrangements for conducting the test and increasing their response rate within the year. Payments will also be made based on trusts' results for a similar question in the NHS Staff Survey.

However you look at it, that's a lot of emphasis on one question. Fred Reichheld, the US customer loyalty consultant responsible for the Net Promoter Score (the inspiration for the test) has described it as 'the ultimate question' and 'the one number you need to grow'.

But is one question enough to evaluate the complex package of transactions and relationships that determine people's experiences of healthcare? Surely not. Likewise, it's difficult to see how answers to that question, in isolation, could possibly drive improvement. Knowing whether someone would recommend your service might tell you about their loyalty to or liking of it, but it doesn't tell you what they liked or disliked or how things could be improved. For that you need more information, more specific questions. You need the capacity to analyse responses and identify themes and priorities and therein lies the gap between the Friends and Family Test as a tool for payment and a tool for improvement.

It follows that the Friends and Family Test cannot, in and of itself, be expected to improve standards of care; indeed we would be naive to imagine that there might be any 'one number' that could.

The Department of Health acknowledge this in guidance on the Friends and Family Test. Organisations are encouraged to use follow-up questions and to drive cultural change. These questions are to be determined locally, as is the method for administering the test. This is critical: it's up to providers to work out how they will use the friends and family test as part of improvement: the onus is on them to decide their own level of engagement.

The best and most ambitious organisations, the ones already trying to live the NHS Plan's decade-old commitment to 'put patients at the heart of care', will see an opportunity. They will go beyond the requirements of the test, using a range of specific, actionable questions; they will use consistent, robust methods; they will make attentiveness to patient experience part of the organisational culture from ward to board. The worst organisations will simply tick the box.

6 February 2013

⇨ The above information is reprinted with kind permission from the Health Foundation. Please visit www.health.org.uk for further information.

'This can't go on' – NHS chiefs urge new debate on health service reforms

An unprecedented crisis is approaching, say the health service's most senior figures.

By Oliver Wright

Hospitals are 'staring down the barrel' of having to cut the jobs of doctors and nurses – actions that could lead to another Mid Staffordshire scandal – unless the NHS radically reforms, the organisation's head warns today.

In a stark assessment of the perilous state of NHS finances, Sir David Nicholson said the health service faced a £30 billion black hole in its finances by the end of the decade because of rising demand.

And he predicted that unless politicians and the public accepted the need to shut and centralise services such as accident and emergency care, cardiac surgery and maternity units, the NHS would no longer be able to cope with demand. Sir David was backed in his remarks by the Medical Director of the NHS, Sir Bruce Keogh, and the Chief Nursing Officer, Jane Cummings.

They called for a 'national conversation' about how to reform the NHS and called for politicians to be honest with the public about what needed to be done.

'What we're really worried about is an approach that would muddle through,' Sir David said. 'It won't. 75 per cent of all the money spent by hospitals is on staff. [We're] looking down the barrel of reducing staffing on wards and that is just not acceptable.'

Asked if that could lead to another scandal similar to that which contributed to the unnecessary deaths of hundreds of patients at Mid Staffs, he replied: 'That is exactly the position.'

> **'Staff and patients say repeatedly we are not providing the best possible care'**

The comments by the three most senior figures in the NHS underline the growing frustration in the organisation at the slow pace of change in reconfiguring NHS services.

While senior politicians accept the need to merge services, when individual hospitals are affected they lead to a barrage of local protests – which often delay plans for months and sometimes years as they are fought through the courts.

Sir David and Sir Bruce argue that specialised services – such as paediatric cardiac surgery, stoke and cancer services – are best if they are centralised in fewer, more experienced units.

'Sir David Nicholson said the health service faced a £30 billion black hole in its finances by the end of the decade because of rising demand'

Sir David warned that ministers – who have to approve all such changes – had to act in the long-term interests of the whole NHS and not short-term political considerations.

'The current regulatory process around those changes is very slow and we need to talk to the Government about how we streamline that because those changes need to happen and happen rapidly,' he said. 'More importantly we need to have a conversation with patients about the necessity to make that happen.'

But he added: 'If a political manifesto does not say that service change is absolutely essential and that you need to concentrate and centralise services – it will not be being straightforward with the British people.'

He also hinted at a new shake-up of primary care, with smaller GP surgeries being forced to merge with other practices where they could provide a greater range of services in the community. This is also likely to meet fierce opposition as it will almost certainly mean patients having to travel further to see their local GP.

Sir Bruce said that patients needed to be aware of the true picture facing the health service. 'The NHS is caught in a triple pincer of rapidly escalating demand, rapidly escalating cost and restrained resources,' he said.

'And all of that is against a background of increasing expectations of better quality care with the principles of the NHS maintained. So that is such a complicated issue. As guardians of the NHS purse we have a duty to ensure we get the best value for the taxpayer.'

Jane Cummings, the Chief Nursing Officer, said even at the moment care was not good enough in certain parts of the country.

If Sir David, who is to retire next year following criticisms of his handling of the Mid Staffs crisis, gets his way it is likely to result in the downgrading of services currently provided by district general hospitals around the country.

They are unlikely to be closed altogether – but will merge services with other local hospitals meaning patients will have to go further to be treated.

But Sir David insisted it was the only way to provide consistent high-quality care in an age of effectively frozen budget.

'The nature and scale of the challenges that we face are so great that we really do have to have a much more radical view about the way we are going to [change],' he said. 'The general approach will be specialisation and concentration in a smaller number of organisations. That is inevitably the consequence.'

Mike Farrar, head of the NHS Confederation, which represents hospital managers, said the Government needed the 'courage and willingness' to challenge how health services were structured.

'NHS England is right to call for an honest and realistic debate between NHS staff, the public and politicians about what needs to change. When that debate has been had, it is crucial that those in charge of the NHS make the changes a reality.'

Chris Ham, chief executive of the health think-tank The King's Fund, added: 'The significant financial and service pressures facing the NHS and social care will continue for some time yet, so it will be important to be honest with the public about the implications of this in the run-up to the next general election and beyond.'

Straight talk: what they say

Sir David Nicholson (NHS chief executive) 'Every year from now on we have to find £4 billion-£6 billion of savings, to deal with new demand.'

Sir Bruce Keogh (NHS Medical Director) 'The NHS is caught in a triple pincer of escalating demand, escalating costs and restrained resources.'

Jane Cummings (NHS Chief Nursing Officer) 'Staff and patients say repeatedly we are not providing the best possible care.'

Patients face treatment rationing

Patients are having their access to some treatments restricted by one in seven of the Government's new clinic commissioning groups, new research suggests today.

The groups were set up by ministers to replace primary care trusts as part of the Government's health reforms. Led by GPs, they have responsibility for deciding what treatments to offer their patients on the NHS.

But an investigation for the *BMJ* found that some CCGs have tightened the thresholds for access to 'low priority' surgery such as hernia and joint problems. Others have introduced new systems to restrict the flow of patients being sent to hospital.

Eight CCGs across north-west London added new restrictions for nasal surgery and a new general cosmetic policy, but also removed restrictions for several procedures including asymptomatic gall stones and caesarean section for non-medical reasons.

11 July 2013

⇨ The above information is reprinted with kind permission from *The Independent*. Please visit www.independent.co.uk for further information.

The practical, spin-free guide to funding the NHS

The NHS needs another 'significant shake-up' as it faces a £30 billion shortfall. But we need to challenge the marketisers' myths.

By Jacky Davis

Today, Sir David Nicholson, who has presided over the disastrous dismantling of the NHS over the past three years, casually lobbed another bomb at the battle-weary service and its staff. The NHS is apparently facing a £30 billion funding shortfall and needs yet another 'significant shake-up'. The assumption follows that we can't afford the service, and the radio phone-in lines are already buzzing with answers to the inevitable question: what can we cut to save the NHS?

This is the wrong question, and falls straight into the Government's trap. Their position is that the NHS is unsustainable, that 'we can't carry on like this'. But those who have watched the NHS brought to its knees by the Coalition have questions to ask, and some solutions to propose that do not involve cuts or payments for service. For that is surely where this Government wants this conversation to end up: the NHS is unsustainable. This is a convenient myth to explain the next myth, that 'things can't go on like this'. The fact is that it is not a given that changing demographics and new drugs necessarily lead to accelerated costs. We must challenge the myths and the figures.

So, where can we save money that would not involve cutting services, already being rationed by hard-pressed clinical commissioning groups (CCGs)? Well, the market in healthcare has taken transaction costs from 6% to about 16% (an estimate, as the Government won't tell us the figures). That's £10 billion a year wasted on marketising the NHS – an experiment which has already proved an expensive failure, as daily headlines confirm. So end the market in healthcare, with GPs having to tender for all services and hospitals criticised for anti-competitive behaviour for attempted mergers.

Want more savings? One London hospital is rumoured to be spending £4 million a year on management consultants. Multiply that across the country, and we can save millions by eliminating the people who steal your watch and sell you the time of day.

Want more? Stop using the private sector, which is neither cheaper nor innovative. Policing them is proving expensive and ultimately impossible. And if you want yet further savings, end the expensive PFI programmes which are crippling hospitals.

What about those expensive health tourists? Forget them, and concentrate on the big stuff. So-called health tourism is estimated to cost between £12 million and £200 million a year, certainly less than 0.2% of the NHS budget. This is pure distraction politics and a sop to Ukip – look over there at those people abusing the NHS, don't look over here at these politicians wrecking it.

Where can we find the money to pay for a service that almost everyone bar the private sector and the politicians wants to remain comprehensive and free at the point of need? Avoid think-tank suggestions about top-ups and insurance, the slippery slope which will carry us away from the founding principles of the NHS. The current way of funding the service has been repeatedly shown to be the most cost-effective and fairest. If we cut the waste and the NHS still needs more money, we just need the political will to raise it. Deal with tax avoidance and evasion, calculated to cost the country up to £70 billion a year, enough to pay for over half the cost of the NHS. Join 11 other EU countries in adopting the Tobin tax, and assign the extra billions raised to the NHS. And if this is not enough, what do you think the public would prefer: a decent health service or Trident?

Finally the big question. Why has the NHS, in the space of three years, gone from being a popular, cost-effective and efficient service, to one that is constantly in the headlines for all the wrong reasons? Could it be that the last significant shake-up has been a disaster and that more of the same might finish off the patient? Don't let's get caught up in the Government's strategy – run the service down, starve it of funds and then claim it has failed and needs yet another massive shake-up, helped by a good dose of the private sector. That's one remedy that we should avoid at all costs.

11 July 2013

⇨ The above information is reprinted with kind permission from *The Guardian*. Please visit www.guardian.co.uk for further information.

NHS @ 65: the NHS cannot do it alone

By Jeremy Taylor

We are in danger of losing our collective nerve over the future of the NHS. In 1948, in the midst of austerity and post-war national exhaustion, Britain created a comprehensive health service which offered care to those who needed it regardless of their means.

It was a courageous idea whose time had come and it made compelling economic, political and social sense. It still does.

In 2013 our far richer country can and should continue to embrace Aneurin Bevan's vision. Of course we face very different health challenges to those of 1948. We live longer; there are more people with disabilities and long-term conditions; there are more very old people. More healthcare is delivered to more and more people. It has become eye-wateringly expensive.

Those, by the way, are largely the fruits of success: decades of rising prosperity and advances in public health, medicine, surgery, pharmacology and technology. Many millions of people have cause to be thankful.

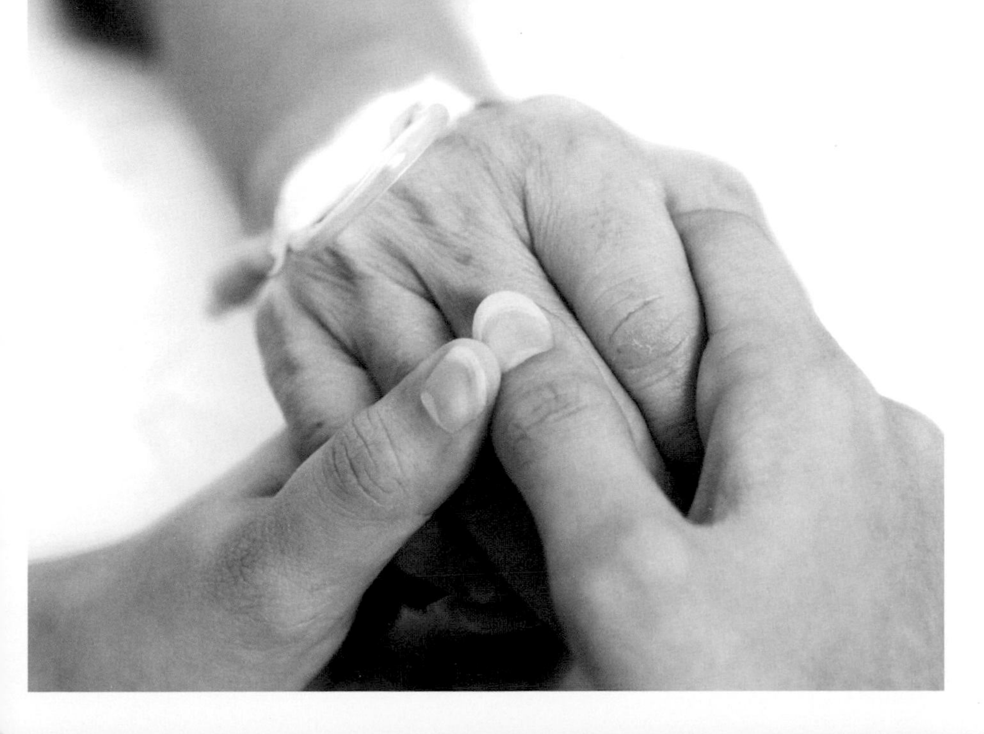

The NHS, as so vividly highlighted in the opening ceremony for the 2012 Olympics, has become woven into our national myth. Opinion polls consistently show it to be popular and well supported.

And yet in policy-making circles the prevailing mood in 2013 is one of gloom. People fret about 'rising demand' and the 'burden' of chronic disease. Hand-wringing about the sustainability of A&E services is the latest fashion as I write.

A scandal in one hospital in Stafford has prompted an unending spasm of inquiries, reviews and navel-gazing about the capacity of the entire NHS to deliver care safely and with compassion.

It has become fashionable to blame patients and the public for profligate use of the NHS. We are eating, drinking and slobbing ourselves to early graves at the taxpayers' expense, failing to 'self-care'; wasting GPs' time; and rolling up to A&E with trivial complaints.

And in this current economic slump it is becoming fashionable, for the first time since the 1980s, to question whether Bevan's settlement – a comprehensive service, free at the point of use – is sustainable and affordable.

Through a mixture of defeatism, lazy thinking and, in the case of some, malign intent, we are in danger of sleepwalking towards dismantling the NHS. Of course there is a lot that needs change and improvement. In ten years' time, a functioning NHS will need coordinated out-of-hospital services for the very old; it will need patients who are informed, engaged and when necessary stroppy; and it will need a more social and less medical, less pharmaceutical model of care.

Before 1948, the great scandal was that your healthcare depended on the size of your wallet. In 2013, the enduring scandal is that the quality and length of your life depend on your postcode. To remove the appalling inequities in health that we have allowed to persist and worsen will need action on many fronts.

The NHS cannot do it alone, but without a comprehensive health service, free at the point of use, we will never get there.

This is an extract from Jeremy Taylor's contribution to the Nuffield Trust publication: The wisdom of the crowd: 65 views of the NHS at 65. The collection of essays was published on Thursday 4 July 2013.

12 July 2013

⇨ The above information is reprinted with kind permission from Nuffield Trust. Please visit www.nuffieldtrust.org.uk/blog/nhs-65-cannot-do-it-alone for further information.

NHS rationing: we need honest politicians to tackle the taboos

By Julia Manning

I've just taken part in a discussion on BBC Radio Kent on the emotive topic of IVF on the NHS. No one can deny, including myself from personal experience, that trying to conceive for some couples is an emotional rollercoaster. The current concern in Kent from infertility consultants is that new guidelines will reduce the availability of IVF to couples in Kent. Before we dismiss this with a 'they would say that, wouldn't they', it is vital to look at the bigger picture.

There are two interconnected big taboos on which politicians owe it to the public to open up the debate, but which most seem to regard as the third rail. The first taboo is being honest about NHS funding. The second is deciding what the NHS covers. Demand for healthcare always has and always will outweigh supply. How many times have we heard politicians say that the NHS has, and always will be 'free at the point of demand', and will provide the 'best' healthcare? It's not true. We are victims of our own success: research and innovation have yielded ever more treatments, techniques and interventions leading to greater public demand, raised expectations and an increase in longevity, (the latter resulting in our being more susceptible to diseases of old age such as dementia and age-related macular degeneration). For many, glasses, medicines, dentistry, wheelchairs, certain specialised drugs are items that you either pay for or can contribute to. If someone wants the best focusing lens implant when they need their cataracts removed, they can't have it. It's not available on the NHS. Nor could they have the latest prosthetic robotic arm if they lost their own in a car accident. As a system of limited resources, it is both totally disingenuous and illogical to promise that the NHS will provide the best of everything.

The projected funding gap for the NHS by 2021/2022 is of up to £54 billion if funding is held flat in real terms, which in the face of the bigger economic picture, and healthcare to date having been ring-fenced, seems a realistic scenario. We cannot divorce the NHS from the national economic reality. We are still drowning in debt; only Greece, The Netherlands, Portugal and Cyprus currently have more private debt (excluding the banking system) than us, and combined UK private and public debt (again excluding the balance sheets of City banks) reached a record of 298% of GDP at the end of last year, higher than the Eurozone average of 268%. To put this in further perspective, at the end of the second world war in 1946, UK debt was 250% of GDP. Added to this, the number of people aged over 65 is estimated to increase by 51% between 2010 and 2030, and the number of people over 85 will double over the same period. We are living way beyond our means, and that includes our tax funding of health.

Part of what has driven this spending is the second taboo: not all conditions that we are able to treat should truly be classified as 'illness' or 'disease'. More and more of us are being turned into patients when our 'condition' is just a variation of human normality. Researchers writing in the *BMJ* last year described us as being 'over-dosed, over-treated and over-diagnosed'. On the one hand we have increased diagnosis, or what is known as 'diagnostic drift': screening programmes that detect early cancers that will never cause symptoms or death; tiny 'abnormalities' picked up by sensitive diagnostic technologies that will never develop; the widening of criteria for being given a diagnosis and genetic testing that gives us a very dubious 'risk' rating, both of which can cause anxiety and possibly lifelong testing and treatments for no benefit.

At the NHS we realise not everyone can get full medical care. We now have a way to make sure no-one misses out: Will you get 100% coverage or just 25%?

Step right up and play...
The NHS Wheel of Fortune!

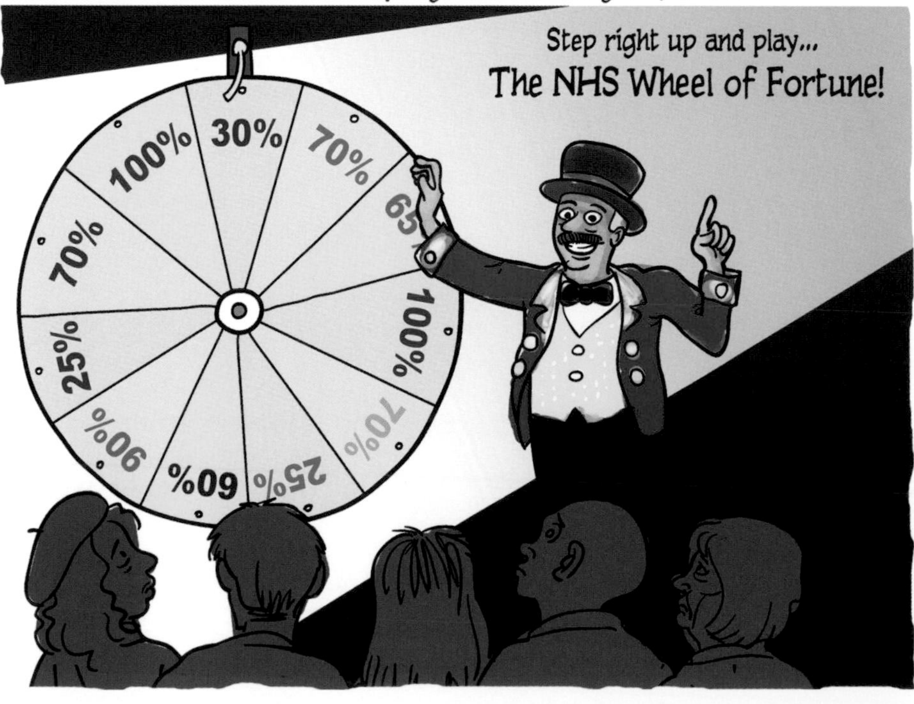

On the other we have an ever increasing number of differences, what were once regarded normal human variation, now labelled as medical conditions. Witness the recent controversy around the American DSM-V bible of mental disorders which includes sadness, shyness, distress and (as do previous editions) also admits 'the difficulties inherent in drawing a precise distinction between normality and psychopathology'. Infertility, the sensitive subject covered in this morning's radio programme, is a relatively common difference between adults. Yes we have medical treatment, and undoubtedly it is a clinical 'want', but a clinical 'need' on which we should be spending tax-payers money? (And I have to mention here the 80,000 children in care and thousands of babies waiting for adoption; it's not the case that you can never have a family.) I am sure someone could make a good 'anxiety' case for having their teeth whitened on the NHS, but we don't fund this, even though they could claim their discoloured teeth are ruining their confidence and life-chances.

There will be many different opinions, but the point I am making is that we need an honest public discussion: we can't afford everything, so what do we guarantee will remain free at the point of delivery? There is an appetite and willingness to spend our own money on our bodies, as demonstrated by the £2.3 billion Britons spent on cosmetic procedures in 2009 (it could be nearer £4 billion now), and the £500 million already spent privately on IVF, as well as other private procedures and consultations. I am not saying this will be easy, or painless, but we owe it to those with serious illness now and in the future the certainty that their needs will be met. And to those feeling that they are facing a postcode lottery for whatever reason, to have the uncertainty removed and know exactly what they can expect from the NHS, no matter where they live. It's high time to tackle these taboos.

11 June 2013

⇨ The above information is reprinted with kind permission from 2020 Health. Please visit 2020health.wordpress.com or www.2020health.org/2020health for further information.

One in two do not trust the NHS

Majorities of all parties say NHS staff should be able to publicly speak out about problems with services – and a slim majority of the public do not trust the NHS to be open and honest about services and standards of care

Yesterday the outgoing chief executive of the NHS, Sir David Nicholson, stood before the Public Accounts Committee to explain his failure to declare payoffs to the sum of £2 million for staff leaving the NHS, which the Committee suspects were used as 'gagging orders' to silence staff wanting to speak out about problems with NHS services. Mr Nicholson denies any cover up, and claims the responsibility for declaring secret payoffs to the Treasury had passed to the Department of Health on the day he took up his post.

Today new YouGov research reveals that slightly more than half (51%) of British adults do not trust the NHS to be open and honest about its services and standards of care. That is compared to 41% who do trust the health service. Labour voters are the only party group to trust the NHS more than they distrust it on the issue, however this is by a very small margin (48% to 45%).

The majority of British adults also oppose the silencing of NHS staff: 56% say 'NHS Staff who find problems with services should be able to publically speak out about them to alert the public and make sure the issue is properly dealt with', while under a third (32%) believe that 'staff who find problems with services should raise them internally where they can be better dealt with and do not cause public alarm or damage confidence in health services.'

What is more, the majority opposed to NHS gagging is made up of supporters of every party: 56% of Conservatives, 61% of Labour voters, 57% of Lib Dems and 67% of UKIP supporters.

Sir David Nicholson was forced to stand down in May over his involvement in the Mid Staffordshire Trust scandal, when the health authority he was in charge of caused the death of between 400 and 1,200 patients by neglect.

Prior to his resignation, a March YouGov survey found that 64% of the public thought that Sir Nicholson should resign.

13 June 2013

⇨ The above information is reprinted with kind permission from YouGov. Please visit www.yougov.co.uk for further information.

Key facts

- ⇨ Since its launch in 1948, the NHS has grown to become the world's largest publicly funded health service. (page 1)
- ⇨ The NHS employs more than 1.7 million people. Of those, just under half are clinically qualified, including, 39,780 general practitioners (GPs), 370,327 nurses, 18,687 ambulance staff and 105,711 hospital and community health service (HCHS) medical and dental staff. (page 1)
- ⇨ The NHS deals with over one million patients every 36 hours. (page 1)
- ⇨ In 1991, 57 NHS Trusts are established to make the service more responsive to the user at a local level. (page 3)
- ⇨ In 1998 NHS Direct launches. This is a nurse-led advice service provides people with 24-hour health advice over the phone. (page 3)
- ⇨ In January 2011, 11.1% of the UK population had private medical insurance. (page 5)
- ⇨ Private hospitals generated revenues of around £3.8 billion in 2010. (page 5)
- ⇨ NHS income from treating private patients in 2011 was £445 million. (page 5)
- ⇨ Hip and knee replacements cost an average of £10,000 each, while MRI scans cost from £600. (page 6)
- ⇨ It is estimated that the NHS performs 250,000 operations each year on patients with private medical insurance, costing a total of £359 million. In addition to which, £609 million is spent on emergency medical treatment. (page 7)
- ⇨ 73% consider the NHS to be one of the UK's greatest achievements. (page 7)
- ⇨ 41% of people in the UK think that the health service as it exists today is unlikely to last until 2020. (page 7)
- ⇨ 53% of people would pay for private healthcare if they could afford it. (page 7)
- ⇨ The monitoring report from the King's Fund showed that in the final quarter of 2012/2013, 5.9 per cent of patients (313,000 people) waited for four hours or longer in A&E – the highest level since 2004. (page 17)
- ⇨ 63 per cent of NHS staff said that if a friend or relative needed treatment they would be happy with the standard of care provided by their organisation. This figure is unchanged from that in the 2011 survey. (page 18)
- ⇨ 15 per cent of NHS staff reported experiencing physical violence from patients, their relatives or other members of the public in the previous 12 months and 30% of all staff report that they experienced bullying, harassment and abuse from patients, their relatives or other members of the public in the previous 12 months. (page 18)
- ⇨ Just under two-thirds of incidents of physical violence and 44% of bullying, harassment and abuse cases were reported. (page 18)
- ⇨ When asked if the healthcare system in Britain needed any changes, over half (55 per cent) said that 'a few changes' are needed, and another third (32 per cent) that the NHS requires 'many changes'. Only five per cent said that no change is necessary – which is also the proportion who maintain that the service 'needs to be changed completely'. (page 20)
- ⇨ The Health and Social Care Act, which became law after a tortuous passage through Parliament, is expected to cost the taxpayer between £1.5 billion and £1.6 billion to implement. (page 29)
- ⇨ So-called health tourism is estimated to cost between £12 million and £200 million a year. (page 36)
- ⇨ £2.3 billion Britons spent on cosmetic procedures in 2009 (it could be nearer £4 billion now), and the £500 million already spent privately on IVF, as well as other private procedures and consultations. (page 39)
- ⇨ YouGov research reveals that slightly more than half (51%) of British adults do not trust the NHS to be open and honest about its services and standards of care. (page 39)

Glossary

A&E
The Accident and Emergency department in an NHS hopsital provides emergency medical care.

Friends and Family Test
From April 2013, all patients treated in NHS wards or A&E departments will be asked on leaving whether they would recommend that department to their friends and family. The Government hope that this measure will help them to guage the standard of treatment in NHS hospitals and also help people make decisions about where they want their medical care to be provided. Results are available on the NHS website.

Health and Social Care Act 2012
The biggest change to the NHS since it was very first started. Came into force in April 2013.

Health insurance/private medical insurance
Although UK citizens are entitled to free care via the NHS, many opt to pay into a private medical insurance policy so that they can choose where they are treated and receive a higher standard of care in more luxurious surroundings.

Health tourism
Foreign visitors who come to the UK so that they can claim free medical treatment that might not be available in their own country.

Francis Report
The nickname of the Mid Staffordshire NHS Foundation Trust inquiry. Robert Francis, QC found that patients under the care of the Mid Staffordshire NHS Foundation Trust were 'routinely neglected by a Trust that was preoccupied with cost cutting, targets and processes and which lost sight of its fundamental responsibility to provide safe care.

Liverpool Care Pathway (LCP)
Introduced as a palliative care measure for terminally ill patients the LCP was intended to be a way to ease the suffering of those who were in their final days. However, the LCP is now being withdrawn after media controversy which claimed that hospitals were employing the LCP with elderly patients without consent in order to meet financial targets.

NHS
The National Health Service provides free medical care to citizens of England, Scotland, Wales and Northern Ireland.

NHS Direct
24 hour medical advice, provided by the NHS, available online and via telephone service.

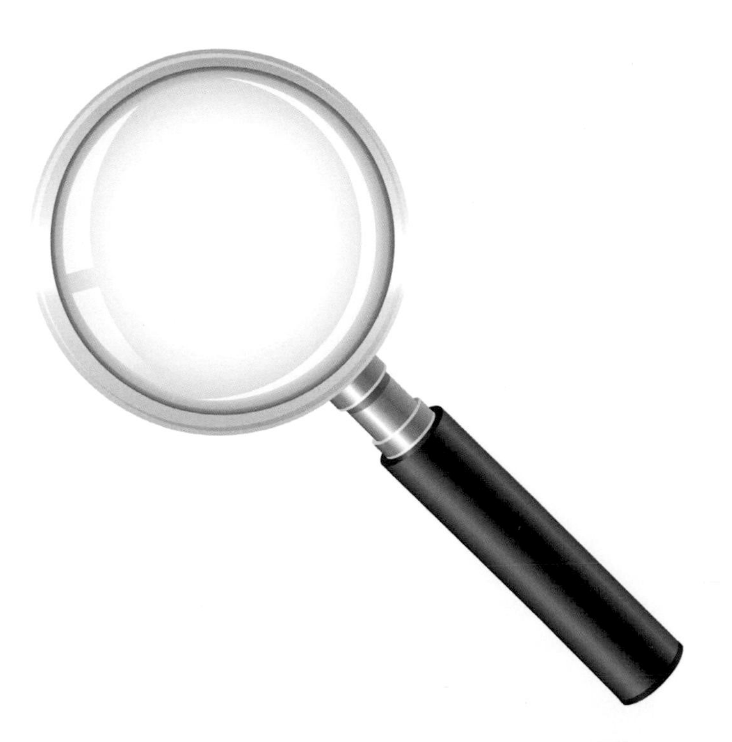

Assignments

1. Imagine that you have been asked to do a presentation to a group of foreign medical students, explaining the history of the NHS and the way it works now. With a partner create a PowerPoint presentation and try to include pictures, statistics or even videos to make it engaging and memorable.

2. Choose an illustration from this book. What do you think the artist was trying to achieve? Did he/she succeed? Write a few notes and then draw your own version.

3. Look at the *History of the NHS in England* timeline on pages three, four and five. Using the NHS Choices website, do some research to see if there are any points that have been omitted from the timeline and create a new version using the things you think are most important.

4. Choose one point from the *NHS in England timeline* on pages three, four and five and research it further. Write an article exploring your chosen point from the timeline.

5. Design an advice guide for people considering whether to purchase a private medical insurance policy.

6. Research the healthcare system of another European country and write a report comparing it to the NHS.

7. Design a poster that celebrates the NHS and its 65th birthday.

8. Using the information from this book create a table that demonstrates both good and bad points about the NHS.

9. Look at the graphs throughout this book and use them to help you create a questionnaire that will be distributed throughout your local community to help gauge public opinion about the NHS. Distribute your questionnaire to as many people as you can and create a report, including graphs and tables, to demonstrate your results.

10. Research the Liverpool Care Pathway and write an article for your local newspaper exploring the controversy surrounding this protocol.

11. Read *Healthcare in Britain: is there a problem and what needs to change?* on page 19. In pairs discuss what you believe are the key points. Create a bullet point list and share with the rest of your class.

12. 'Foreigners should not be allowed to claim treatment on the NHS.' Stage a class debate in which half of your argue in favour of this notion and half argue against it.

13. Write an information guide that will be distributed at your local GPs surgery explaining the Health and Social Care Act 2012 and the changes that followed.

14. Do you think the Friends and Family Test will improve the quality of care in the NHS? Discuss in small groups.

15. What treatment do you think should be covered by the NHS? Discuss with a partner and create a list of the treatments or care options that you think the NHS should pay for, and a list of things you think it should not pay for. For example, should cosmetic surgery be available on the NHS? What about weight loss surgery? When you've created your list feedback to the rest of your class and talk about how you made your decisions. Did you find it easy or difficult?

16. Every day for one week read a selection of national newspapers (online or in print) and write down all the headlines you see about the NHS. At the end of the week tally up the good headlines and the bad headlines. Does the NHS receive more good press or bad? Do you think this is justified? Bring in some examples of the articles you read and discuss with your class.

17. Do you know anyone who is a Doctor or a Nurse? If you do, ask them about their different experiences of the NHS and write a few paragraphs summarising what they say.

18. Imagine that you are the son/daughter of an elderly patient who you believe has not been receiving adequate care at your local NHS hospital. Write a letter to your local MP explaining the situation and what you think needs to be done to improve NHS care for the elderly.

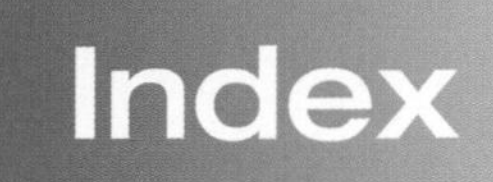

Index

Acknowledgements

While every care has been taken to trace and acknowledge copyright, the publisher tenders its apology for any accidental infringement or where copyright has proved untraceable.

Illustrations:

Pages 1 & 30: Don Hatcher; pages 8 & 23: Simon Kneebone; pages 24 & 38: Angelo Madrid.

Images:

All images are sourced from iStock, Morguefile or SXC, except where specifically acknowledged otherwise.

Additional acknowledgements:

Editorial on behalf of Independence Educational Publishers by Cara Acred.

With thanks to the Independence team: Mary Chapman, Sandra Dennis, Christina Hughes, Jackie Staines and Jan Sunderland.

Cara Acred

Cambridge

September 2013